IF YOUR EYES
COULD TALK

IF YOUR EYES COULD TALK

THEY WOULD TELL OF THEIR INVOLVEMENT IN
READING PROBLEMS, ANXIETY, HEAD TRAUMA,
FATIGUE, AND MUCH MORE...

D. TODD WYLIE, OD, FCOVD

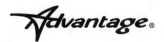

Published by Advantage, Charleston, South Carolina.
Member of Advantage Media Group.

ADVANTAGE is a registered trademark and the Advantage colophon is a trademark of Advantage Media Group, Inc.

Printed in the United States of America.

ISBN: 978-1-59932-779-2
LCCN: 2017940151

Cover design by Katie Biondo.

Advantage Media Group is proud to be a part of the Tree Neutral® program. Tree Neutral offsets the number of trees consumed in the production and printing of this book by taking proactive steps such as planting trees in direct proportion to the number of trees used to print books. To learn more about Tree Neutral, please visit **www.treeneutral.com.**

Advantage Media Group is a publisher of business, self-improvement, and professional development books. We help entrepreneurs, business leaders, and professionals share their Stories, Passion, and Knowledge to help others Learn & Grow. Do you have a manuscript or book idea that you would like us to consider for publishing? Please visit **advantagefamily.com** or call **1.866.775.1696.**

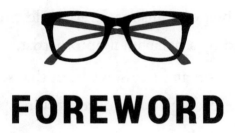

FOREWORD

When I graduated from my surgical ophthalmology residency, I felt I had all the skills to save anyone with vision problems. I felt that eye disease was something to "cut" and put back together again. I felt that the eyes were like a faulty car engine that could be corrected by taking out old parts and replacing them with new ones. After fifteen years of a very successful surgical practice, I began to see that our eyes and vision were much more than a mechanical system for vision. As one of the leading alternative eye doctors practicing for over twenty years, I wonder if there could be more to vision and eyesight.

I have known Dr. Todd Wylie for over ten years and am very grateful that he has written a book on a missing element of vision. In his exciting new book, *If Your Eyes Could Talk*, he reveals that our eyes are much more than a sensory organ for sight.

Dr. Wylie not only tells you how your eyes are speaking to you but also what you can do to correct the problems they are contributing to such as reading problems, anxiety, fatigue, and many more.

One important chapter addresses vision and learning disabilities. There are thousands of children who have been labeled slow learners and poor readers when, in fact, the problem is in their eyes. I am not talking about getting reading glasses but learning through specific eye exercises to help the eyes function properly. I have seen students' lives transformed when they develop proper use of their eye muscles. Every child who has learning difficulties should be evaluated by a behavioral optometrist.

In the chapter on vision and stress, we learn that stress affects simple day-to-day vision tasks, like reading and comprehension, sports, and even driving.

A chapter on syntonic light therapy shows a quick way to reduce stress and improve vision function. Read about a remarkable way that a ten-minute light treatment can help to reduce stress and to improve vision function. Light therapy is becoming more and more accepted for treating pain and depression but also is remarkable for improving reading skills, comprehension, and general well-being.

Dr. Wylie discusses a relatively new area of optometry called prism lenses. These are specialized lenses that are unlike the traditional lenses in your eyeglasses. These lenses can be useful for those with walking and balance problems. Read about people who had amazing transformations using these prism lenses.

There is a chapter on a commonly undiagnosed problem—traumatic brain injury—that affects vision and mental health. You will learn methods of diagnoses and treatments using light and specialized lenses that could greatly help affected patients.

The book concludes with good advice on nutrition, visual hygiene, and ways to improve not only eye health but also overall health.

This book should be an essential part of your library, especially if you are interested in having optimal health. Your eyes do speak to you, and it is important that you listen to them.

Edward C. Kondrot, MD, MD(H), DHt, FCSO
Host of *Healthy Vision* Talk Radio

TABLE OF CONTENTS

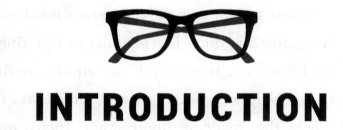

INTRODUCTION

My earliest memory of reading is in my aunt and uncle's house. I remember looking at a book and the excitement of realizing the marks on the page were starting to turn into words, and those were starting to turn into pictures in my head. I remember the excitement of starting to figure things out. I remember just marveling at that.

I started enjoying reading more and more. In grade school, I was pretty much a bookworm. I can remember going down to the library every day one summer to check out another ten-plus books. My mom was very kind to take me to the library daily. I would bring home a stack of books, read them, and go back the next day for another stack. I think I read over two hundred books that summer.

My next memory is in fourth grade. I remember my teacher sending me to the principal's office, and I could not figure out what I had done wrong.

The school nurse was there. She checked my eyesight, and then sent a note home with me to tell my mom to take me to the eye doctor. That point began my journey with being nearsighted (seeing blurry distance vision). From that point on, I would go to the eye doctor and get a new prescription every year. That would be it for about a year, and then I would be blurry again and go back. I continued doing that through freshman year of high school.

When going to the eye doctor, I remember my mom not being excited with the six frames to choose from for my glasses selection. That was my first time going to an optometrist. Not only did they have a much wider selection, but I remember them checking other parts besides just putting drops in my eyes and seeing what I could see. They were doing some interesting tests where I was trying to line things up with both eyes, and some tests of how the eyes were working. Initially, that made an impression. "There's more to an eye exam than just looking at the eye chart and getting eye drops."

Sophomore year in high school, we took an anatomy and physiology class. Bob Bastion, our science teacher, was a tremendous teacher. Everyone loved him. On Fridays, we would spend most of the class watching slides from when he was in the Air Force in Alaska. I am sure everyone in our sophomore class planned on going to Alaska some time in their life. My wife and I were able to do that for our twenty-fifth wedding anniversary. It was absolutely wonderful.

In the anatomy and physiology class, one of the assignments was to write a paper on a science-related profession. I started thinking. Our family, the prior year, had joined the small sailing club in Klamath Falls, Oregon. One of the top sailboat racers on the lake was an optometrist. He also played wonderful trombone. Since that was my instrument, I thought, "This person seems to know what's important in life, so I think I'll do an article on optometry."

As I researched it, I realized there was no blood, and there were normal working hours. Since I had been wearing glasses since fourth grade, I thought optometry sounded like a good profession. I had talked to my pediatrician about going to medical school, but he discouraged me from doing that and encouraged me to pursue optometry.

I graduated in 1975 and "set sail" to Pacific University in Forest Grove, Oregon. I went there as an undergraduate to try to improve the odds of getting into the graduate program of optometry at Pacific. It is the only optometry school in the Northwest. Since it was a five-hour drive from Klamath Falls, that worked out very well.

My studies for undergraduate went along pretty well. I was not a straight-A student, but I was getting very good grades. Things were going nicely until my junior year when things started to change. I started taking organic chemistry, a prerequisite for optometry school. Chemistry has never been my strength, so I knew it would be a little bit rough.

I noticed that during that term, after five or ten minutes of reading, I would start to get drowsy and fall asleep. I thought, "I need to get more rest. It's college." I got more rest, and I would read and start falling asleep again. My reading comprehension also decreased. I would be reading along, and pretty soon I would realize, "I don't remember what I've just been reading."

Chemistry was not going well during this time. I was failing. I can still remember my week of doom quite vividly because I was reading text. I would read a paragraph, stop, and think, "What did it say?" I couldn't remember. I went back and read it six times in a row. I still could not bring up what I had just read.

For this week of chemistry, I knew I had to get the upcoming test. I kept track and studied thirty hours that week for the organic chemistry test. I took the test. When I got the results back, I was devastated. Out of those thirty hours of studying that week, I scored an impressive eight points out of fifty. That was not a good hours-per-point ratio for studying. I knew I was in trouble.

I scheduled an appointment to go to the optometry clinic to have my eyes checked. I had my eye exam by the optometric student intern, and he let me know the good news. My glasses prescription had not changed a bit. I could still see 20/20 in each eye. However, he then went on to demonstrate that my ability to converge or aim eyes inward was horrible.

That was my first introduction to behavioral optometry and vision therapy. At that point, I did not know that optometrists did anything above and beyond eyeglasses and contact lenses. However, I started immediately doing some vision training to teach my brain to get better at coordinating my eyes. Thankfully, because the condition had popped up so quickly, it took six to eight weeks of training procedures that I would do in the clinic and in my dorm room for a few minutes a day.

After the six to eight weeks, I noticed that my reading comprehension had returned. Literally by God's grace, I was given a C in chemistry. I remember Dr. Curry. I am positive he gave me a C because he knew my heart was in optometry because I still do not see how I could have passed that class. Thankfully, I did.

I was then accepted to optometry school after my junior year of undergraduate. Freshman year, we had a January term where we took one class for only three weeks. This class was taught by a dear optometrist from Portland, Oregon, Tole Greenstein, who gave me a further introduction into the history of behavioral optometry and inspired me to learn more.

One of our professors, Dr. William Ludlam, was a very dynamic instructor who was passionate about behavioral optometry. He was a genius. He had grown up in New York and helped establish the Optometric Center in New York, or SUNY. When he was married and had children, Pacific University was able to woo him westward for an improved place to raise his family. He helped establish the vision therapy department at Pacific University. He was incredibly driven, and his enthusiasm was contagious.

During my freshman year, after taking the introduction to vision therapy class on learning disabilities from Dr. Ludlam, I asked if I could observe in his clinic. That began a wonderful three and a half years of riding in with Dr. Ludlam two to three times a week after class for the initial year and a half of observing his patients several hours a week. He had patients coming to see him from Alaska to Los Angeles. It was fascinating. Beginning my junior year of undergraduate, he asked if I would be interested in starting to do vision therapy with his patients. I began to get hands-on training in doing the therapy.

I was able to spend over 1,400 hours observing and working in Dr. Ludlam's vision therapy office over those three and a half years. The experience was truly incredible. I was seeing the changes in people's lives that would occur on a weekly basis.

I moved to Spokane in 1982 after graduating from optometry school, and I have been doing vision therapy ever since. As you will find out later in this book, it has been a continued journey of learning more and more amazing aspects about the visual system.

In 1993, I learned about syntonics, or colored light therapy. In 2003, I had the pleasure of meeting Rick Collier, OD, from Allen, Texas, who provided earth-shattering information and research he gleaned from many disciplines that has impacted hundreds of patients with a particular type of lens, a yoked prism, or as Dr. Collier called it, a binary lens, because it changes the timing of light to the brain.

I look back and am humbled by the people who have touched my life in learning about many ways to work with the incredible design of the visual system, and what wide-ranging effects it can have on people's lives.

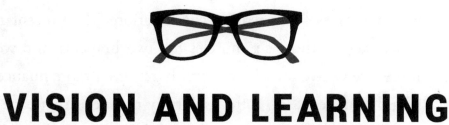

VISION AND LEARNING DISABILITIES

If your eyes see 20/20, can they still interfere with the ability to learn to read or read to learn? Most definitely they can, and 20/20 is only one very small measurement of the entire visual system. We have five times the sensory input to the brain from the visual system of any other sense that we have.

In the vast majority of the states, the school "vision screening" involves looking at an eye chart twenty feet away. How much of the time is spent in a classroom looking twenty feet away when studying?

Dr. Herman Snellen developed the eye chart back in 1862 when he was looking for ways to help measure the ability of troops going into the Civil War. Unfortunately, technology for school eye screenings has not quite kept up with the times. We are now doing so much more sustained near-point close work, yet the school screening does little to pick up people who are having difficulties seeing near print. Moreover, over 95 percent of people with vision-related learning disabilities see 20/20, so eyesight is not the problem.

We take our eyes for granted. When one starts looking at the complexity of the visual system, it truly is remarkable that anyone learns to read. The eyes are the only organs in the body that have different components being controlled by two different nervous systems coordinating at the same time.

The central nervous system controls our eye movements. There are six muscles going to each eye that require coordination. More recent research has realized that each of those six muscles has two branches and would be considered more like twelve muscles per eye. It gets even more nuanced from that. Dr. Richard Bruenech, PhD, from Norway mentions that each muscle actually has four components. Ongoing research continues to show more and more complexity of our visual system.

The eye muscles of the body are the strongest muscles for what they need to do of any muscle in our body. Our eye is a one-ounce object, and the eye muscles are one hundred to two hundred times stronger than they need to be.

When we look at the accuracy of movements, the eye has the ability to move the very smallest of degrees. Our leg muscles have one nerve fiber going to about one thousand muscle fibers. In comparison, the eye has the lowest nerve to muscle ratio of any muscles in our body. It is a one-to-twelve ratio with one nerve for every twelve muscle fibers allowing for very small, precise eye movements.

With such a fine controlled system, why would people have problems keeping their place with reading? Why would they tend to skip words or get to the end of the line and lose their place when they go to look to the next line? It is because of the interaction with the other components of the visual system where problems can arise.

When we are beginning readers, we are still learning how to improve accuracy of eye movement. Tracing large letters in kindergarten and first grade is part of what helps develop eye movements. Over thirty years ago, researchers took infrared monitoring devices that would record where a person fixates or points their eyes when shown different objects. Since an angled line provides more information than a straight line, fixations tended more often toward angles.

When researchers would show people a picture, every person had a particular scan path or order in which their eyes moved about the objects. Though in general, people's eye movements gave a similar pattern, the order in which each person moved their eyes was unique. What was of further interest is when they continued to repeat the process, after a few repetitions, suddenly 35 percent of the time when people would look at the picture, their eyes no longer moved.

Researchers concluded that part of the memory of an object initially is involved with the eye movements that lay down a scan path or order of movement. When a person goes to look at the object again, the eyes start repeating and replicating the scan path to help identify the object. Later, it can be more of an internal shift of attention not requiring eye movements.

Suppose during the scan process someone does not have the ability to accurately control his eyes. When he looks at an object he makes the first scan path. Due to poor control, when he looks at the same object he then makes a slightly different scan path. As his brain starts reviewing, it realizes, "This is a novel scan path, so I don't know what this object is.

This very likely accounts for some of the frustration in the learning-to-read process when a person sees a new word; he learns what it is, and then in the next paragraph, he cannot recall what that word was that he just saw. Maybe on another day when he is more rested and he has improved eye movements, he can identify the word. Then later on in the day when he is more fatigued, he has less efficiency and less accuracy, and he is no longer able to replicate the previous scan path. Once again, he "doesn't know" the word.

Another part of the visual system that is crucial for doing near-point work is our accommodative or focusing system. This changes the shape of the lens in our eye in order to focus the light precisely on the retina so we see clearly.

The eye is definitely not like a camera. A camera takes a picture, and all of the picture should be in focus. With the eye, only the straight-ahead vision common from the macular or pinpoint of sharpest sight is capable of providing clarity. From a 180-degree retina, it is the central one degree that has enough light receptors to provide clear detail as well as color. It is also that central one degree that causes the focusing system to respond. Once again, the person's ability to accurately point his macula at the proper target in the proper order is crucial for the focusing system as well.

The third main component involving the eyes for reading is the ability for the eyes to point or converge at the reading material. This aiming ability is absolutely crucial for efficient reading. We have all seen people who have an eye that wanders out or crosses. That is a strabismus, or eye deviation. In many of their cases, reading is not hugely interfered with because they have already learned how to turn off or suppress the central vision in the eye that is deviated. However, they can have difficulties in other areas of day-to-day life, like depth perception and night driving difficulties.

This ability to easily align the eyes for reading is absolutely essential for the ability to read quickly as well as influence a person's ability to comprehend what he is reading. I described my personal experience in the introduction to this book when I experienced a convergence insufficiency, or difficulty aiming eyes inward for reading. Another imbalance is a convergence excess or a tendency for the eyes to cross or over aim. There can also be a tendency for one eye to want to aim slightly higher than the other. Any of these imbalances can be devastating for the reading process.

Over twenty-five years ago at the Pacific University College of Optometry, Dr. Bill Ludlam supervised a study involving forty-eight third-year optometry students. These would have been people with six to seven years of college education.

They made two pairs of glasses. One pair was essentially window glass and had no power in it. The other pair had nine units of prism positioned so it would give the simulation of someone who had a convergence excess or tendency for their eyes to over aim. To compensate for this, the person would have to spend energy aiming their eyes outward from the target in order to keep clear and single vision. Prior to the test, they confirmed there was no blurring and no doubling at any time during the reading.

They gave the forty-eight optometry students four equally weighted sections of the California Achievement Test for reading speed and comprehension. They did two tests with each pair of glasses, and the participants did not know which pair of glasses they were looking through.

The results of the study were that forty out of forty-eight of the grad students had a statistically significant drop in reading speed and reading comprehension when they were wearing the pair that made them have to spend extra energy to keep their eyes aligned. This interference with reading comprehension occurred with no blurring and no doubling of vision.

This once again shows how subtle vision imbalances can be because they do not have anything to do with clarity of sight but have all to do with the amount of energy and effort it takes to make the different components of the visual system function.

I use this demonstration in my office frequently when I have parents who have brought in their son or daughter with reading difficulties. About three out of four times, I am able to give the parent a "vision-related" learning problem where suddenly they now have difficulty with reading speed, keeping their place with reading, or comprehending what they are reading, or they will feel significant visual strain or eyes aching while reading. Suddenly, the parent has a great deal of empathy for his or her child as far as the amount of hard work he or she is spending in the reading process.

Because convergence insufficiency is such a frequently found deficit among those with vision-related learning disabilities, there has been some very well-done research funded by the National Eye Institute on more random-ized clinical trials of treatments for symptomatic convergence insufficiency in children.[1] You can go to the website www.ConvergenceInsufficiency.org to see this study as well as others that found that the most effective treatment for this vision disorder was vision therapy in a doctor's office along with home reinforcement.

Treatment for vision-related learning disabilities can run the gamut. Simple reading glasses that help balance the aiming and focusing system and allow for greatly improved performance are one option. Another option is the yoked prism lenses described in another chapter in this book.

Syntonic light therapy is described in a separate chapter of this book. It is often part of the treatment as well. In addition, vision therapy, more accu-rately described as vision neurorehabilitation, procedures are quite effective in helping a person's brain learn how to gain better control and coordination over the various parts of the visual system. As a person develops improved control with less effort they can then learn how to utilize the information the eyes are taking in.

Vision perception is utilizing the information coming in through our eyes and applying that to our previous memory. Accurate visual perception provides a clear, understandable picture of where we are in space and synchro-nizes with hearing, balance, and body awareness or proprioception.

---

1 *Archives of Ophthalmology*, 126(10), October 2008.

The good news is that there is treatment and hope for children or adults with vision-related learning disabilities. It is trainable at any time. A number of years ago, I had a husband and wife who brought their ten-year-old son in for evaluation. He was very bright but was having significant difficulties in keeping his place when reading. He would frequently reread the same line. He had a difficult time concentrating and paying attention when doing his schoolwork. He definitely had a visual imbalance, and we began doing the vision neurorehabilitation.

About two weeks later, his father came in for an exam. He was a CPA. He told me he was working roughly eighty hours a week just trying to keep up with the paperwork. He would go home every night absolutely exhausted and found it difficult to spend time with his family because his eyes and head hurt, and he was so fatigued. Upon further questioning, he said reading had always been difficult. He said he had literally blocked out most of his high school memories because he had to work so hard for school. Boy, talk about someone who picked a profession that was not conducive to a poorly operating visual system!

Nevertheless, it was found that he indeed had a vision-related learning disability just like his son. The two of them, father and son, began doing the rehabilitation. I will never forget the visit when the father came in and was describing how, for the first time in his life, he was enjoying reading.

It was also the first time in his life he was able to appreciate 3D vision. He was driving along one of the streets in Spokane Valley, and all of a sudden the world "popped 3D." It took him totally by surprise. He pulled off to the side of the road and just looked around in awe, seeing the added dimension he was now able to perceive. He had no idea that the world really looked three-dimensional. As he continued on, he was becoming more and more efficient with reading and doing his work. By the end of the therapy he was able to get more work done in forty hours a week than he had been able to do in an eighty hour week. He, his wife, and son were thrilled with the increased family time they could enjoy each week.

To see if you, your child, or loved one might have a vision-related learning disability, please see the attached checklist or go to my website, www.DrWylie. com, for an online checklist. Please do not hesitate to investigate. It can make a difference for a lifetime.

VISUAL EFFICIENCY CHECKLIST

Any of the following symptoms may indicate a functional vision problem. Please check all the symptoms that occur and calculate the total. Compare to the scoring criteria at the end of the list to determine if a functional vision evaluation is recommended.

If you would like to schedule an evaluation, please make note of your score as you will need this when scheduling.

Check all that apply:

- O Skip lines while reading or copying
- O Lose your place while reading or copying
- O Skip words while reading or copying
- O Substitute words while reading or copying
- O Reread words or lines
- O Reverse letters, numbers, or words
- O Use a finger or marker to keep place while reading/writing
- O Read very slowly
- O Have poor reading comprehension (unless read to)
- O Have difficulty remembering what has been read
- O Hold your head too close when reading/writing (within 7-8")
- O Squint, close, or cover one eye while reading

O   Have unusual posture/head tilt when reading/writing

O   Have headaches following intense reading/computer work

O   Have eyes that hurt or feel tired after close work

O   Feel unusually tired after completing a visual task

O   Have double vision

O   Notice vision blurs at distance when looking up from near work

O   Have crooked or poorly spaced writing

O   Notice the print goes in and out of focus

O   The print appears to "move" or "wiggle" at times

O   Have poor spelling skills

O   Notice that letters or lines "run together" or words "jump" when reading

O   Misalign letters or numbers

O   Make errors when copying

O   Have difficulty tracking moving objects

O   Notice unusual clumsiness, poor concentration

O   Have difficulty with sports involving good hand-eye coordination

O   Have an eye that turns in or out

O   See more clearly with one eye than the other

O   Feel sleepy while reading

O   Dislike tasks requiring sustained concentration

O   Avoid near tasks such as reading

O   Confuse right and left directions

O   Become restless when working at a desk

O   Tend to lose awareness of surroundings when concentrating

O   Find you must "feel" things to see them

O   Experience carsickness, worse in the backseat than the front seat

O   Experience unusual blinking

- Experience unusual eye rubbing
- Experience dry eyes
- Experience watery eyes
- Experience red eyes
- Have eyes that are bothered by light

SCORE:

CRITERIA:

- 15-20 points total = Possible functional vision problems
- 21-30 points total = Probable functional vision problems
- Over 30 points total = Definite functional vision problems

- 15+ total points = Functional vision evaluation recommended

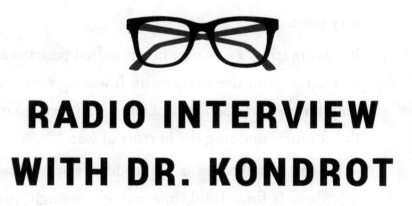

RADIO INTERVIEW WITH DR. KONDROT

Vision and Stress

Welcome to *Healthy Vision*, the talk radio show to help you conquer your vision loss. Dr. Edward Kondrot is a board-certified ophthalmologist and homeopathic doctor, author of four best-selling books. *Healthy Vision* is dedicated to bringing you the latest information for a lifetime of healthy sight and to help you conquer your eye problems.

Dr. Kondrot: Welcome, everyone. This is your host, Dr. Edward Kondrot. I just got back from a two-week medical mission in Vietnam. My wife and I were on a sixteen-hour flight today coming back from Vietnam. This medical mission was sponsored by Vets with a Mission, a group of Vietnam veterans who go back to Vietnam every year and give back to the people.

It was a very moving experience for me working as an eye doctor in some of the poorest remote areas in Vietnam between Da Nang and the DMZ where much of the battle took place. These people receive absolutely no medical care. There is no Medicaid or welfare system in Vietnam. They're very poor.

It was amazing. I saw over one hundred patients a day, and I had to use primitive equipment. It was a great experience not only for me but also for all the vets that went to give back to the country, undoing the horrors of war.

With me this evening is Dr. Todd Wylie who has been on this show before. Todd, interestingly enough, just got back from Israel where he was on a pilgrimage, a kind of biblical tour. Both of us have returned from missions, so to speak. Dr. Wylie, it's great to have you on the show.

Dr. Wylie: Thank you, Dr. Kondrot. Thank you again for your service to humanity in Vietnam and helping out those folks. It's so wonderful you're able to help with that and touch hundreds of lives every day.

Dr. Kondrot: It's a little bit of a different way of practicing. Normally, I take about an hour for my initial examination. In the jungle, I didn't have the team. Every five minutes I was seeing two or three patients.

I had to relearn my skills for retinoscopy. That's a device eye doctors use. By just shining a light in the eye, you can determine whether or not the person needs glasses, whether they have a cataract, or whether there's a problem. I was brought back to my old tools.

I wish I'd had a connection with you. I could probably use some retinoscopy pointers. It's a way we can measure someone for glasses without them responding to which is better, one or two.

You and I have a lot to talk about. I'm very excited with our topic this evening, which may seem like an unusual topic. It's anxiety and our visual system. This is not what people would think. It's not the anxiety people get when they're losing their vision or when they have a cataract. This is anxiety that comes about with an imbalance in the visual system. Is this correct?

Dr. Wylie: Yes. It's something we don't think is even related. We think, "Our eyes are for seeing." If they can see 20/20 and they're healthy, that's often as far as some people will go thinking the eyes are involved with the body. It's literally the tip of the iceberg.

There are so many connections to different parts of the body from the visual system. Literally half the nerves from our eye to our brain have nothing to do with eyesight. Over 70 percent of our brain receives input from the eyes, but they're not necessarily seeing connections. That's what we'll talk about this hour.

We'll look at different things for people to ponder on and be aware of. Maybe something eye-related can be contributing to some of their difficulties. There are also some nice ways of treating this system. Treating the visual system can help with cognitive processes and ease anxiety in many cases.

Dr. Kondrot: The first thing that comes to my mind is the wrong way the medical system is treating this. For anybody who has anxiety and visual problems and goes to see a doctor, the first question the medical doctor will ask is, "Have you seen your eye doctor?" They'll usually say, "Yes, I did. He said it has nothing to do with my eyes." The medical doctor will then prescribe Prozac, Valium, or some type of medication. They're not even touching the problem, which is causing a major disservice to the patient.

How else is the medical field not addressing this? For that matter, a lot of our colleagues are eye doctors. Are they missing this connection? Let's talk a little bit about that.

Dr. Wylie: Let me give one example of a sixty-nine-year-old patient who came from Seattle to Spokane a couple of years ago. He initially heard about my office from his niece.

She had been going to college, but then she dropped out because of poor reading comprehension. She was failing, and then she came into the office. Through some unique lenses that influenced the timing of light to the brain, and also some light therapy, which helps with balancing the fight-or-flight nervous system, she was able to go back to college and was on the honor roll.

Her uncle heard about this. His whole life, he'd only been able to read for ten minutes at a time before he'd have to put the book down because he couldn't remember or comprehend what he was reading. He also mentioned that he'd had major anxiety his whole life. He had actually taught himself self-hypnosis so that when he was in crowds he would not freak out.

He came over to Spokane and had a "wow" with this particular type of lens that changes the timing of light to the midbrain. We sent him home with some light therapy procedures. He came back six weeks later. I asked how things were going. He said, "I'm now reading two to three hours a clip, two to three times a day. I'm devouring books." I asked him, "How's your anxiety these days?" He said, "Wait a minute. There hasn't been any."

In getting the visual system working more efficiently, it really had an impact on his life. He was doing the best he could to make up for lost time in reading, and he was enjoying it.

Dr. Kondrot: Folks, we have a most interesting topic this evening: anxiety and our eyes. This is overlooked by many eye doctors. By addressing this problem and understanding the underlying cause and what it's doing to the neurological system, amazing results can be achieved. With me is Dr. Todd Wylie.

We're coming up to a break. When we come back, we'll go into more detail about how to diagnose this problem and some of the amazing treatments Dr. Wylie is offering in his office. You're listening to *Healthy Vision*, and we'll be right back after this break.

Welcome back to *Healthy Vision*. This is your host, Dr. Kondrot. We have a fascinating topic: anxiety and our eyes. During the commercial break, Dr. Wylie and I were talking about how there is a two-way street. Stress can cause problems with our eyes. On the other hand, problems with our eyes can lead to stress. It's up to the eye doctor to determine the causative factor. I wonder if you could talk a little bit about this situation.

Dr. Wylie: It may be acute stress. The classic example would be if you look down the road and there is a charging rhinoceros coming at you. That doesn't happen too often in the United States. Maybe a variation on the theme for Dr. Kondrot would be a water buffalo or something in Vietnam.

If the person, all of a sudden, is in a fight-or-flight survival mode, there are a number of physiological effects our body does for survival. One of them is sending blood to our limbs so we can run faster and jump higher. There's also a decrease in stomach acid production because when we're running for our lives, that's not the best time to digest a meal.

Visually, our pupils will dilate to let more light in. Our focusing system will tend to focus far away to look at the threat. Eyes will posture outward, which is also for looking far away. We'll also get varying amounts of a tunneling of vision because we're so focused on the threat.

The police academy actually teaches police cadets that when they're in a really stressful situation, they should try to remember to use a head scan because there's physiologically a tunneling of peripheral vision.

With the acute stress of a charging rhinoceros, we hopefully jump over the wall and get away from the threat of being trampled! Then our fight-or-flight nervous system calms down.

Sometimes that doesn't happen. If somebody is in a car wreck or some kind of trauma, and the results of that trauma persist for days, weeks, or months, the body can get habituated or stuck in this fight-or-flight mode. There's also chronic day-to-day stress where adrenaline is being released and the body is on sympathetic nervous system activation. You get the same physiological effects either way.

So much of our world requires sustained up-close work on computers and reading. If our visual system is physiologically set for decreased focusing at near and the eyes are postured outward, this is the opposite of what you need to do when you go to read. You have to aim your eyes inward. Right there, even though your eyes physiologically are trying to posture outward, your demand for near-point is making your eyes go inward. It's like two rams butting heads as far as the nervous systems fighting each other. That ramps up stress.

That tunneling of peripheral vision can also happen. It's not something wrong with the person's vision, like a stroke causing a loss of peripheral vision due to damage. It's a functional compression of the visual field. That tunneling can get stuck and persist for months, even years.

All these problems can have huge ramifications for a person's tendency to get overwhelmed or overloaded by sensory input when shopping or driving. They have a hard time on the freeway. They don't want to change lanes. Maybe they're wandering through a fabric store or hardware store, and all the visual input can literally be overwhelming.

People start to realize, "I feel anxious." They start having anxiety, and it can be from the physiological effects from the visual system. If somebody just doesn't have great coordination and control, the huge amount of energy required to operate the different parts of the visual system will cause stress, which activates the sympathetic fight-or-flight nervous system.

You can have it from either direction. It can be stress-induced causing a visual problem or poor eye coordination to begin with causing stress, which then results in anxiety and impact on day-to-day function.

Dr. Kondrot: You described some symptoms. Immediately in my mind, I related it to some people I know and some situations in my life when I had it. Does the general public or medical profession refer to this state? Have they given it a name? Is it, "That person is stressed out. They're not functioning well?" How does the general medical profession refer to this?

Dr. Wylie: Typically they will say, "That's called anxiety or some OCD tendencies."

Dr. Kondrot: It's anxiety of unknown origin probably. They really don't know what causes it. They don't know what to do. It's normally a pharmaceutical approach, which in most cases doesn't take care of the underlying problem.

I like the idea where you mentioned ADD, attention deficit disorder, or learning disorders. Many children have these phenomena. I think a lot of adults have it too. When I was in Vietnam, a lot of vets there had a lot of trauma. They were not able to read or function properly. They don't realize that the stress is affecting the visual system, which is affecting their ability to read.

When you see somebody like this come into your office, is there a quick way to diagnose this condition? What do you do as an eye doctor to confirm that they do have this anxiety state tied into their eyes?

Dr. Wylie: There are a number of different measurements. One part is during the eye examination itself and looking at how easily a person is able to converge or aim their eyes inward. It's not only measuring their ability to do that but also watching and listening for how much effort it's taking.

It's also watching their pupils. With the sympathetic fight-or-flight nervous system tending to dilate pupils, you can shine a light directly into the eye of people with this condition, and instead of constricting and staying constricted or smaller, we might see a pulse, but then it blows back open to virtually the same size whether the light was on it or not. That's another clue.

We'll also do a different type of peripheral vision test rather than the push-the-button kind we're used to from going to the eye doctor that just checks pathway integrity. This is more of a moving target. How soon can somebody tell there's something different going on in his or her peripheral vision? That's where we can measure these different amounts of functional tunneling of vision, which is also very helpful for explaining why things are frustrating and overwhelming.

Some of the kids or adults with ADD keep moving around and scanning around. It appears they're not paying attention. If they happen to have this functional tunneling of vision, it's as if you cup your hands around your eyes. If that's all they can take in at a time, some of them are scanning their eyes around to maintain manual awareness of their peripheral surroundings. It looks like they're not paying attention, but they're having to manually pay attention in an extremely inefficient manner.

Dr. Kondrot: We're coming up to another break. This is really interesting. The bottom line is that the diagnosis can be made very quickly without a lot of very sophisticated tests like brain scans or x-rays. It's simply looking at the pupil and observing the eye muscle. When we come back, we're going to be talking about simple treatments that can correct this problem. You don't want to miss this. We'll be right back after the break.

Welcome back to *Healthy Vision*. This is your host, Dr. Edward Kondrot. With me is Dr. Todd Wylie. We're talking about a very interesting topic: anxiety and our eyes. Doing certain treatments on your eyes can dramatically reduce your anxiety and stress. That seems hard to believe.

Before we go into these simple treatments Dr. Wylie does in his office, Dr. Wylie is coming out with a book dealing with all of this. He feels so strongly that the public has to know more that he's putting all this together in a book. I want to congratulate you, Dr. Wylie, for putting all this together in a book. Tell us a little bit about the book.

Dr. Wylie: The title will be *If Your Eyes Could Talk.* If your eyes could really talk, they would be able to tell how they may contribute to anxiety, stress overload, learning disabilities, and symptoms associated with head trauma. In the book, I will look at some of our behaviors and discuss how a poorly coordinated visual system could contribute to these behaviors.

What if a number of different day-to-day tasks are not going so well, such as poor reading ability and poor comprehension, difficulties in sports, even problems with driving comfortably without effort? If this happens day after day, over time could your eyes actually affect your personality? Maybe somebody gets super stressed out and wants to avoid people and crowds, or their kids bother them because they make noise. It can have significant impacts on interfamily relationships if the visual system is not helping but is hindering or interfering with life.

Dr. Kondrot: It sounds like it's going to be a great book. You have an offer. You're recruiting people to ask questions and contribute to the book. They can get on your mailing list and find out what you're doing. The feedback from people out there who have these eye problems would be great. If you have a question for Dr. Wylie, sign up on his email list and keep up to date on the progress of this book. Can you give us the contact information for how they can get a hold of you?

Dr. Wylie: Ideally, email would be the best. It's nice and short. It's my initials for Donald Todd Wylie, so it's DTW@CET.com. My office phone number in Spokane is (509) 535-5855. Email would be best. That way we can address the issues and answer questions.

There's also a questionnaire related to stress, anxiety, and the visual system. We'd be happy to send it out if you want to see if some of the things where you think, "That's the way I am" maybe don't have to be that way. There's a self-scoring list that gives an idea of the probability of the visual system contributing to some of the anxiety issues.

Dr. Kondrot:	That's a great bonus. You can go through that checklist to see if you fit into one of those categories.
	I had to smile when you said people might think, "That's just me. I've been that way all my life." Folks, you don't have to be that way all your life. Maybe you're locked in to a neurological state that a simple treatment can help.
	Dr. Wylie, let's talk about some of the simple yet very amazing treatments that can turn this condition around.
Dr. Wylie:	There is a combination of things. Some of it that is extremely helpful is syntonics or light therapy, which is using specific colors or frequencies of light to stimulate different parts of the nervous system in the body toward balance. I've been doing that since 1993, and I literally cannot imagine practicing a day of optometry without using syntonics.
	Unfortunately, there are just a few hundred of us in the country who use it. It's one of the best-kept secrets out there. Anything we can do to help spread the word of some other options that are non-pharmaceutical but really help get to the underlying root of how to balance things without the side effect of drugs is amazing. Physiological research within the last ten years is exploding with learning about the effects light has on the body.
Dr. Kondrot:	This light treatment is very simple. All you do is select a certain color filter, depending on the state of the person's autonomic nervous system. They just look at it for ten minutes, and the effects are dramatic.
Dr. Wylie:	Yes. It's incredible how our system is receptive to light.

Dr. Kondrot: I have to give a personal testimonial. About ten years ago, I was invited to speak at the College of Syntonics on homeopathy. I flew to Albuquerque cross country. Of course, I was stressed. During the meeting, they did some cursory evaluation like you talked about, looking at my pupils and the way they dilated. They told me I was in an anxiety state. I was. After flying, you have jet lag and you're not thinking clearly.

It just blew my mind when after a ten-minute light treatment, my entire state shifted. Not only did my state shift at that particular moment. I had a problem going into department stores or shopping malls with a lot of florescent lights. I would walk into a room and have a mild anxiety state. My sensory system was overwhelmed. After that syntonic light treatment, it caused a balance in my body.

That convinced me over ten years ago to use syntonic light in my practice treating serious chronic diseases like glaucoma and macular degeneration, which light therapy does help.

I'll put you on the spot, Dr. Wylie. Maybe you could explain how light therapy can treat anxiety. What is the mechanism?

Dr. Wylie: We talked about our fight-or-flight nervous system. One of the physiological responses is the tunneling of peripheral vision. That's one of the hallmark symptoms of the fight-or-flight nervous system being stuck on. We can use different colors of light, which start to balance the system. As it becomes more balanced, the peripheral vision starts to open up. Literally a person can take in more information per unit of time.

It's like putting more RAM or desktop memory into a computer. It can handle more information without freezing up. That's what happens to us with anxiety. With more "RAM" in our system, we can handle the day-to-day input and deal with it rather than it jamming us up.

Light bio photons, which are life-produced particles of light, are operating in every cell of our body at the DNA level. It's incredibly complex how our body utilizes light. We can use different colors or frequencies to help direct and balance the body's use of light, and it has effects physiologically.

Dr. Kondrot: We're coming up to another break. When we come back, Dr. Wylie is going to give us more information about this remarkable treatment, and maybe some other things he does. We'll be right back after this break.

Welcome back to *Healthy Vision*. Those of you who are interested in Dr. Wylie's book, the number to call is (509) 535-5855. That's his office number to get more information on his new book and the treatments that he does. You can also email him at DTW@CET.com. As a bonus, he's going to be sending a checklist you can go through to see if you suffer from this disorder and to see if some of these treatments can benefit you.

On the break, Dr. Wylie and I were talking about how light therapy is one of the best ways to adjust your body to get rid of jet lag. Right after we're done with this interview, I'm going to do some light therapy. It's simple.

In addition to light therapy, you're doing something else interesting that not that many eye doctors are aware of. It's called yoked prisms. What in the world is that?

Dr. Wylie: A prism basically bends or shifts light. Normally we think of a prism that will take white light and create a rainbow. The ones we use are very small amounts, like one-half, one, two, or three degrees at the most.

In the regular ophthalmic world, sometimes prisms are used for compensatory reasons. If someone has an eye that aims higher, they'll put a prism in so the eye can still be high, but the person's visual system is brought together so they're not seeing double. That's not a yoked prism. That's compensatory.

Yoked means the equal amount of prism, but we orient either up or down. I'm so thankful for the insight from the late Dr. Rick Collier from Allen, Texas. For twenty-five years, he spent a day a week in a medical library reading brain research and biophysics to get background and pull this together for how the prism can affect the timing of light to our brain.

In our midbrain is where the nerves originate that go to our eye muscles for moving around. They also significantly communicate with our inner ear for balance as well as hearing.

There's another connection with proprioception. Those are joint receptors in our ankles, knees, hips, neck, and fingers. Those receptors give our brain an idea of where different body parts are compared to gravity, position, and where they are in space. Our midbrain is the control center of helping us know where we are in space.

The timing of each of those systems—the eye movements, the hearing, the balance, and the body—ideally should be the exact same among all four of those systems. It's four times the speed of the signals for our sight.

There's a whole lot going on from a non-sighted perspective that helps us in day-to-day life. Trauma, ear infections, and different things can throw that timing off because the vision has such a huge input to the midbrain. Seventy percent of the nerves going into the midbrain connect with the eyes in a non-sight connection.

By using the yoked prisms, we can change that timing of light to the brain. For some people, literally instantly it can change their life. It's a therapeutic lens, so the vast majority work their way out of them over time. Unfortunately, there are a few dozen of us in the country who use that type of lens. It can be profound.

I had a sixty-five-year-old gentleman a couple of years ago, a very bright guy, who changed careers. He decided to get more physical and started to unload semitrailers for FedEx. Seven years before I saw him, he was unloading a trailer when there was a chemical spill. He passed out and hit his head on the way down.

When I first saw him, he had been suffering anxiety. In the evening as it started to get darker, his anxiety level would start to go through the roof. If he closed his eyes for more than a second while he was standing, he would fall to the ground. When it got dark, his balance was horrendous and his anxiety was off the charts.

The yoked prisms don't help everybody, but when they do, it's very apparent. In his case, we had him standing up, and when he'd close his eyes, he'd start to fall down. With the particular orientation of the prism lenses, he put them on and could close his eyes and stand there totally stable.

We have a video of him the day before he got the prism glasses where he was trying to walk on his deck at home with one foot in front of the other. He definitely could not have passed the sobriety test at all. He was falling all over himself. Then he had his wife videotape him the day he got the prism glasses. He could walk the line forward and backward with no hesitation. Just changing the timing of light can impact life significantly.

Dr. Kondrot: I think it's really hard to explain what a prism is. When you put a prism in front of your eye, the image jumps a little bit to one side or the other or up and down. It causes a subtle shift. What you're saying is that there's a neurological imbalance. For some reason, light is not sent into the brain properly.

Dr. Wylie: Yes. It's a timing issue.

Dr. Kondrot: Do the prism therapy and light therapy go hand in hand? Do most of the patients you treat need both of these treatments? How do you determine what patients need the prism and what patients need the light?

Dr. Wylie: It depends. We check everybody out to see. Some benefit from both. Sometimes one or the other can make a difference.

One other avenue we utilize is a type of pulsed electromagnetic frequency device. I can't mention the name right now because it's going through Class II certification with the FDA.

33

If you want to contact me personally, I can talk further about it. It has an incredible impact on circulation to the body.

Blood flow to the body is something that also is very detrimentally affected, particularly with chronic stress. This would also impair blood flow to the brain. There is a device specifically targeted for that. NASA has a working agreement with this company to help incorporate the technology in the undergarments for the astronauts because of the issues they have in space with poor circulation.

When we combine that with the light therapy, we've been doing some studies where literally in eight minutes we can make a measurable difference in the person's peripheral vision, which helps with brain fog or the ability to think. That's been another very exciting area of synergistically combining some different treatment modalities that really help one another, and quality of life can be significantly improved.

Dr. Kondrot: Dr. Wylie, we're coming to a close on *Healthy Vision*. I can't believe how quickly the time went. Thanks so much for all your information that you shared with us. Folks, if you want to keep up to date on Dr. Wylie's work, give his office a call at (509) 535-5855 or email DTW@CET.com.

Dr. Wylie, I look forward to your book that's coming out soon. We'll need to have you as a guest on the show once your book is released.

Dr. Wylie: Thank you very much, Dr. Kondrot.

Dr. Kondrot: Folks, you're listening to *Healthy Vision*. This is your host, Dr. Edward Kondrot. To all of you out there, good health and clear vision.

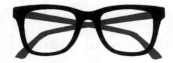

SYNTONICS LIGHT THERAPY

Imagine less anxiety, fewer panic attacks, and less frustration. Imagine an increased feeling of well-being, increased productivity, more energy, and a happier you. In a moment, you will learn about a physical reason that could be a major contributor to the above problems. You will see how a basic understanding of our body's normal mechanisms could be the cause and how to use this same mechanism as a solution, all without drugs.

What if your visual system is part of the problem? What if it is the problem? Though you see fine, the visual system could still be a significant contributor to the above problems.

Stress is taking its toll. Are you stressed out? Have you been through significant trauma in your life? Have you not felt the same since? This is not for someone in a severe crisis with self-harming thoughts. Please contact a mental health professional. If you cannot handle stress the way you used to, please fill out the checklist on page 40 to see how significant the problem is.

As a background, there are two main nervous systems in our body. The parasympathetic is the relax/repair nervous system. It helps with nutritional uptake for the cells and the day-to-day maintenance and repair of our body. The sympathetic is our survival or fight/flight nervous system.

Let's look back at when life was simpler. There were no taxes, no traffic jams, no bagpipes, and no accordions. (Sorry. It's a joke!) Life revolved around survival. Let's say we are on a walk in the jungle. We notice a rhinoceros has spied us and is charging full speed toward us. Exciting and exhilarating? I don't think so.

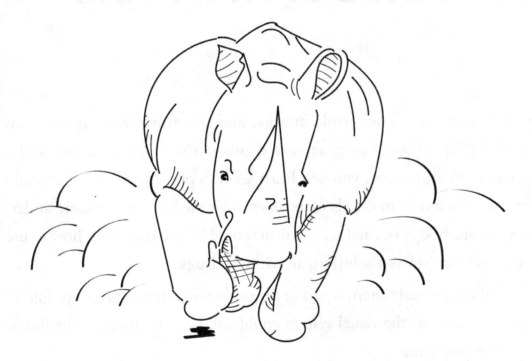

Immediately, our sympathetic fight-or-flight nervous system activates. This causes a number of life-saving changes. Our heart pumps more rapidly. The arteries contract to send blood to our arms and legs so we can run faster and jump higher. Stomach acid production lessens. With a charging rhinoceros coming at us, it is not the time to be digesting a meal.

Visually, there are a great number of physiological occurrences that happen as well, things we have no idea about but that happen automatically. Our eyes posture slightly outward so we can see the threat. Our ability to focus at near decreases because we are looking at the distance threat. Our pupils dilate to allow more light in. Our peripheral vision tunnels down, so the threat is the main object of interest to which we are directing our attention.

This happens with everyone. In police academies, police teach the cadets, when they are in a very stressful situation, to remember to scan with their head because of the tunneled peripheral vision.

All these things happen automatically to increase our survival and avoid the threat. With a charging rhinoceros, we are given the blood flow and nervous system to run faster and jump higher to get away from the rhinoceros.

Once we get away, our heart rate slows. Our blood vessels relax. Our pupils return to normal, and we regain the ability to focus and easily point our eyes to see things up close. Our peripheral vision opens up. The threat is gone. All systems are back to normal. Oh, for those simpler times of life or death.

Seriously, how have things changed? I cannot recall the last patient I had whose life had been on the line due to a charging rhinoceros, but I know many people who are chronically stressed. Day after day, it is stress, stress, stress. How does a chronically stressed person's body respond? It responds the exact same way as with the charging rhinoceros. Our eyes posture outward. Focusing at near is more difficult. Pupils dilate. We get a decrease in stomach acid production. We can also get a tunneling of our peripheral awareness.

What are symptoms associated with these physiological changes? We can have decreased reading speed as well as blurry near vision. We can have eye pain or discomfort when trying to do sustained near-point work. Computers require four times the amount of energy as the written page to look at, so symptoms will show even quicker. Our ability to comprehend and concentrate decreases. We have a harder time maintaining clarity on near-point objects. We have an increased sensitivity to bright light, not to mention the halogen blue driving lights that bother everyone. Lighting in stores is also more bothersome.

From a digestive perspective, we are likely going to have an increased chance of heartburn. Without sufficient stomach acid, our food tends to ferment like a compost heap rather than digest with an increased amount of acid to break the food down so nutrients can be extracted. We will have an increase in tendency to be sensory overwhelmed or overloaded. Along with this is increased frustration. With the tunneling of peripheral vision, we can become more frustrated or fearful when driving.

We can also seem to lose objects we are sure were right next to us. We cannot find them, but then all of a sudden somebody points out, "It's right there next to you." We can also become increasingly startled by people coming into our peripheral vision. Driving on freeways becomes more difficult and often contributes to anxiety. The fast-moving cars increase our frustration. If we dare get on a freeway, there is a tendency to just stay in one lane and avoid lane changes.

I had a patient who drove a delivery truck. During his first visit, he said he felt like he had OCD, obsessive-compulsive disorder. He was very easily frustrated when doing paperwork. It was becoming more difficult for him to complete his tasks at work and on the computer. He also mentioned he had a very strong fear that "I would be in an accident in my delivery truck and not know that I had an accident." The wonderful news is that within just nineteen days, his symptoms were completely gone, and he felt totally comfortable driving even on the narrowest part of his delivery route.

What if there was a way to rebalance the fight-or-flight nervous system as we just talked about with the patient above and help with resolution of the symptoms? What if you could do this in ten minutes a day without drugs? Would you be interested? What is the cost of going day to day with such stress, frustration, and difficulties? What is the cost not only to you but also to those around you?

How can you learn to balance and regain balance in your life? How can this be done without pharmaceuticals and with 100 percent safe treatment? This can be done with different wavelengths or colors of light. How can light do this? It seems too good to be true.

There are amazing biological effects to light. For decades, the ultraviolet lights or bilirubin lights in the hospitals have been used to help infants' livers improve their function. There is also the use of the SAD light for seasonally affected depression. If you want further glimpses of the additional research available, google LLLT and eye and brain. LLLT stands for low-level light therapy. There is a summary of multiple studies about the biological effect of light.

In a nutshell, different wavelengths of light can be used for just a few minutes a day to increasingly nudge different physiological symptoms into balance. The eyes really are the window to the body. Twenty-five percent of our total energy expended each day is used by the visual system. Our brain receives five times the sensory information from the eyes compared to any of our other senses.

There are not that many doctors in the country familiar with syntonics. I am one of the only doctors in Oregon, Washington, Idaho, or Montana who does the syntonic or light therapy. The website www.CollegeOfSyntonic Optometry.com is a good resource for additional information or for looking for a doctor near you.

ADVANCED EYECARE & OPTICAL

Source: Stuart Tessler, OD, www.fightorflighttherapy.com

Could you benefit from Syntonics Light Therapy?

Choose a number from 0-5 that best represents the amount of difficulty, or the severity of the problem you tend to have for each item listed. Don't dwell on any particular question. If you're not sure, go with your gut feeling.

If it varies, indicate how bad a problem it can be. If you are successful at avoiding the problem, indicate how much difficulty you would have if you couldn't avoid it.

0=zero difficulty or problem
1=slight difficulty or problem
2=more than slight difficulty or problem
3=moderate difficulty or problem
4=a lot of difficulty or problem
5=severe difficulty or problem

1. BEHAVIORS

Do you have difficulties or problems with

____ stress

____ mental clarity

____ maintaining your focus

____ organizing your thoughts

____ organizing your life

____ change

____ fatigue or lack of energy

____ feeling frustrated or stuck

____ feeling anxious

____ feeling overwhelmed

____ being easily startled

____ hypersensitivity to sound or light

____ feeling confused or fragmented

____ memory or recall

____ following directions

____ little things that make you frustrated or angry

____ feeling frightened for no apparent reason

____ irritability

____ being overly sensitive or defensive

____ being reactive: "reacting" instead of thoughtfully "responding"

____ feeling impatient	____ crying easily
____ panic attacks	____ persistent or excessive sweating
____ excessive worry	____ depression
____ shallow breathing	____ winter depression SAD (Seasonal Affective Disorder)
____ feeling disoriented	____ seeing your options
____ feeling out of control	____ making decisions
____ feeling "frozen"	____ seeing the "big picture"
____ being overly cautious or hyper-vigilant	____ getting a good night's sleep

____ **TOTAL SECTION 1**

2. DRIVING

Do you tend to be

____ uncomfortable in heavy traffic?

____ uncomfortable when changing lanes?

____ sometimes surprised by cars around or behind you?

Do you tend to

____ bump the curb or other cars while driving or parking?

____ have trouble parking your car straight?

____ have trouble judging distances when driving, parking, or passing other vehicles?

____ find driving a task that requires effort and concentration, rather than relaxing?

____ **TOTAL SECTION 2**

3. CONCENTRATION

____ Do you find it difficult to concentrate on your job, schoolwork, or projects?

____ Do you have any difficulty with concentration and/or comprehension when you read?

____ Do you have eye fatigue that affects your job, schoolwork, or reading enjoyment?

_____ When concentrating, if distracted or interrupted, does it require effort to regain your concentration?

_____ Do you tend to procrastinate?

_____ Do you have difficulty starting projects?

_____ Do you have difficulty completing projects?

_____ Do you have difficulty multi-tasking, usually having to concentrate on tasks individually?

_____ **TOTAL SECTION 3**

4. ORIENTATION

_____ Do you tend to be uncomfortable in crowds and groups?

_____ Would you consider yourself "directionally challenged?"

_____ When you misplace something, do you frequently find it in a place you already looked?

_____ Do you sometimes have difficulty finding an item on a crowded supermarket shelf?

_____ Do you tend to bump into things, trip or miss a curb or stair, or bang your head when ducking under things?

_____ Do you sometimes feel or function as if you have tunnel vision?

_____ Do you tend to be a little clumsy?

_____ Do you experience motion sickness, nausea, or dizziness?

_____ **TOTAL SECTION 4**

5. LIGHTING

_____ Are you bothered by lights or glare?

_____ Do you have trouble with night vision or night driving?

_____ Do fluorescent lights bother you?

_____ **TOTAL SECTION 5**

6. PAIN

_____ Headaches: frequency?

_____ Headaches: severity?

_____ Other chronic physical pain: severity?

_____ **TOTAL SECTION 6**

7. TRAUMA

_____ Have you ever suffered any significant physical, mental, emotional, sexual, birth, medical, or other kind of trauma? (grade: 0=none to 5=severe)

_____ To what degree do you feel these traumas are still causing difficulties in your life today?

_____ **TOTAL SECTION 7**

8. STRESS

_____ On a scale of 1–10, what does your stress level tend to be, with '1' being a laid-back beach bum and '10' being an air traffic controller who is the single mother of three?

_____ **TOTAL SCORE**

How did you do?

There are a total of 350 points possible—most high-functioning individuals score fewer than fifty.

Many people even score thirty or fewer, some even fewer than ten.

If you scored over fifty points, please seriously consider how syntonics light therapy can improve not only your visual processing system but also your overall quality of life.

BINARY LENSES 1

Imagine your child instantly reading more easily. It is possible. I have seen it hundreds of times. Imagine an immediate decrease in reading frustration. We see that in our office on a weekly basis.

In a moment, learn of a test that can be done to immediately improve reading speed and efficiency for some people. Learn how a particular type of a spectacle lens can improve eye movement accuracy and, along with that, gain the benefits of improved fluency, speed, and comprehension of reading. Learn how this discovery has nothing to do with eyesight, nearsightedness, farsightedness, or astigmatism. It is a different use of a type of optics, which has a profound impact on brain function.

THE PROBLEM

Reading is crucial for success in schoolwork and basically for life. Unfortunately for some people, learning to read or reading to learn is very difficult. "I am stupid" is a very common thought of many people with reading difficulties. Thinking "I am stupid" can affect a person's whole life. They can put limitations on themselves that do not have to be there. Because of their experience of having to spend so much energy reading for little gain, one can see how easily that thought becomes a part of them.

What if it is not true? What if looking through a specific type of lens elicited a "Wow!" from the reader as well as anyone listening?

MY STORY

My name is Todd Wylie. I am an optometrist and fellow in the College of Optometrists in Vision Development. I am board certified in vision development. I have been a doctor of optometry in Spokane, Washington, since 1982.

In 2003, I had the absolute life-changing joy of meeting Rick Collier, OD, from Allen, Texas. To honor the memory of Dr. Collier and his groundbreaking work which has profoundly helped thousands of patients, I have entitled these two chapters "Binary Lenses." This was the term he used when describing to me in 2003 how these lenses were different from those that compensate for nearsightedness, farsightedness, or astigmatism. In the next chapter, you will learn about these differences. Before I get into the discoveries Dr. Collier made, let me back up. As Paul Harvey would say, I'll give a little background to the rest of the story.

In 1982, I was fresh out of optometry school. My wife and our five-month-old daughter, Carolyn, moved from Pacific University in Forest Grove, Oregon, up to Spokane, Washington. At the time, the economy was such that inflation was in the double digits. Klamath Falls, being a logging town, had a very high unemployment rate, so we looked for someplace with a more diverse economy and ended up in Spokane.

We met a couple shortly after that. He was a dentist, and his family attended the same church as ours. When they had their first daughter, they had a very rough time. The girl was born a couple of months premature and was in the ICU for two months. During that first year, she almost became a SIDS (sudden infant death syndrome) statistic. One evening, they found her blue and were able to resuscitate her. She survived.

After a few years, our families ended up going to different churches. Around 1998, "for some reason," this family, particularly their daughter, kept coming to mind. I kept wondering how their daughter was doing. I wondered if the early trauma she had gone through had any residual effect on her life. (Please see the syntonics or light therapy chapter as that links in with trauma.) I was wondering whether this young lady would benefit from syntonic therapy if the trauma she had had when she was little was still showing through.

As the thought returned several times, I ended up calling the parents and leaving a message on their recorder. A couple of days later, the mom returned the call. Common courtesy would say you would call the person back. That is where it becomes a little strange because, "for some reason," I would not call the mother back.

This went on for a couple of weeks at least of me just thinking to myself, "You need to call Diane's mom." (The name has been changed.) I would not return her call. I just dropped it. It seemed like about every six months or so for the next couple of years, I would suddenly think, "Not returning a phone call I initiated is one of the rudest things I have ever done to somebody on purpose," but I still would not make the call.

In the summer of 2003, I had a patient that a naturopath in Coeur d'Alene, Idaho, had referred to me for visual evaluation. This patient moved from Dallas, Texas, for several months to work with this naturopath on mold detoxing. The patient had significant visual difficulties. She began doing syntonic light therapy to help with her system. As she was getting ready to move back to Texas, she came in one last time, and I passed on the name of a chiropractic neurologist in Dallas from whom I had taken some courses. It turns out he then referred her to Dr. Rick Collier for evaluation.

In July of 2003, I received a phone call from Dr. Collier. As I answered it, there was a very animated gentleman talking rapidly about this patient and how I could use prism lenses to change the timing of light to her brain. He kept going on and on. I understood about every third word he said, but I could tell he knew a whole lot I had no clue about. I definitely wanted to learn more. I ended up talking to him a second time and asked if he would be willing to come up to Spokane to share what he was learning. We scheduled a time for the middle of September 2003 for Dr. Collier and his wife to spend three days with my staff to show us what he had learned.

About three weeks before Dr. Collier was to arrive, I was working at the office on a Friday morning doing paperwork when the mother of Diane walked into the office. I had not seen her for over ten years. She was referred in by a friend of hers, a patient in my office, to look at Silhouette frames from Europe.

I said, "Hello! How are you? How is your oldest daughter doing?" The lady sat down for a moment and got a little teary-eyed. She said, "Funny you should ask. As we speak, she's finishing the last part of her neuropsych evaluation. For the last four to five years, she has been hallucinating. Any medication makes the hallucinations worse. School is a nightmare." She mentioned that her daughter had no short-term memory and was going to be a senior in a private high school.

Within a moment, the daughter called her mother and said, "Mom, I'm done. Will you come pick me up?" The mother said, "It will be about twenty minutes." She continued to say that her daughter had been tutored every year in math, yet she still could not recite her times tables. Even more alarming was the fact that her parents had not been able to leave her alone one night in eighteen years because she would freak out and could not bear the thought of being separated from her parents overnight. Within two or three minutes, the daughter called back. "Mom, I'm done. Will you pick me up?" not remembering she had made the phone call just a few minutes earlier.

I mentioned to the mother that there was a doctor from Dallas coming in three weeks to show us some very interesting things. Would it be all right if he did an evaluation on her daughter? She said that would be fine. We set the daughter up to see me one week before so I could see what I could see by looking at her visual system.

The week came, and she arrived for the exam. She was nearsighted. Wearing contacts, she was seeing 20/20 in each eye. However, at her reading distance, she had a very poor ability to converge or aim eyes inward. This can most definitely have a significant impact on reading. I know this from personal experience. (See my story in the Introduction.)

Because of the difficulty with her ability to converge, she was intermittently suppressing or turning off central vision in one eye or the other. That is another very detrimental visual deficit that can impact learning. I could tell there were difficulties with Diane's visual system. We also checked her peripheral vision. Surprisingly, that was totally fine.

The next week, she was the first of four patients we had Dr. Collier see when he was up for that first trip. Diane was sitting in the exam room as Dr. Collier came in. My three therapists, the mother, and I were standing back observing. Dr. Collier sat down and asked Diane, "What do you like?" She said, "I like my dog." He said, "Tell me about your dog." She said, "I like my dog. We play. I like my dog. We play. I like my dog. We play." She was stuck. She could not come up with other wording.

Dr. Collier paused and said, "That's fine. I want you to gently rub your thumb and first finger pads against one another back and forth with both hands, and tell me about your dog." Diane was looking at him quizzically but started rubbing her fingers. She said, "I like my dog. We play. I like to go to the park and throw the Frisbee for the dog." She went on for a couple of minutes describing what activities she liked about her dog, meanwhile looking at her fingers, and looking at her mom. We were looking at her fingers, looking at her, and looking at one another. Dr. Collier smiled.

He went on to later explain how reading some research done by the University of Nebraska anesthesia department had given him a clue to have Diane do the finger rub. It certainly has been fascinating on many patients since.

Dr. Collier asked Diane to keep her head straight and watch his finger at reading distance, about a foot off to the side. He said, "Just watch my finger. As I move it in front of your head and I'm passing in front of you, just say 'stop' when it feels like my finger is straight out from the middle of your nose." He did it, and she was watching. It went about eight inches past her nose when she said, "stop." He came across from the other side, and she said "stop" again approximately eight inches to the left of the middle of her nose. This is called a midline shift. It is another clue that her senses are not synchronizing.

He also had her stand up, walk down the hall several steps, turn around, and walk back. We noticed when she was walking that her feet were turned outward. She had kind of a broad duck-walk gait, which is for increasing stability when walking. With a midline shift, she would be feeling that the middle of her was off to the side. This confusion between perception and reality would cause the broad-based walk for added safety and stability.

He then did some other measurements and had us build a trial frame with some prism in front of each eye oriented in a certain vertical position. She put the prism glasses on over her contacts, and he asked her to walk down the hall.

She used the broad duck walk for about two paces. Then her feet went straight, and she continued walking normally. In a couple more paces, she said aloud, "A hallucination tried to come, but it can't." We were all looking at her. She was dumbfounded as she was walking around. Dr. Collier then started asking her math problems, and she started snapping them out.

By this time, almost everyone in the office was crying happy tears. Needless to say, she ended up getting a prescription with the special lens put into the glasses that she would wear over her contacts.

We saw her a week later to begin doing in-office vision therapy and vision rehabilitation. The mom came in with happy tears to explain that her daughter had just written a three-page report. The teacher had asked for only one page. In her life, Diane had never been able to write more than one paragraph on a page.

Diane began vision therapy. It was interesting to note that she did not need the light therapy at all. When we first began working with her, her test of visual perceptual skills showed overall she was in the 9th percentile. Ninety-one people out of one hundred would do better than she would overall on that visual perceptual test.

We continued to work with her. She continued to wear her special lenses. Within a month, her dad mentioned to his wife, "We have two normal daughters." They had wondered if she would ever live independently or get a driver's license. He and his wife went away for four nights on a vacation, and the daughter did completely fine. By February of the next year when we rescored the test of visual perceptual skills, she was in the 99th percentile almost across the board for visual perception. School was so much better. She was reading for pleasure and enjoying life.

That story has an additional cherry on the top and will probably forever rank as our all-time "God gets the glory" story.

It just so happened that that year, the Silhouette frame company, which our patient had referred the mom to us to look at in the first place, was having a contest. "How have Silhouette frames changed your life?" We knew the frames had not changed the daughter's life, but they were instrumental in getting her into the office to receive the help she needed.

We encouraged the mom and daughter to write up a story explaining what had happened. They did not do it. However, the friend who referred them did. She found out that she and her husband had won one of the first prizes, and they were awarded a trip for two to New York City for a Silhouette frame fashion show with all expenses paid.

Because the drawing was done in our office, somebody from our office would get a trip for two to New York to attend the same fashion show with all expenses paid. We put employees' names in the hat. My oldest daughter was working for me at the time. I had her reach in to pull a name out of the hat. It happened to be one of our vision therapists. Desi and her husband ended up getting to go to New York.

During the prior year, Desi herself found that she benefited from these special lenses and had used a Silhouette frame to hold them. In virtually everyone, this type of prism is a therapeutic lens, and over time the patients work their way out of their glasses. Although she did not need them anymore, she took them with her to New York for the fashion show just to wear so she could be part of the ambience.

On the way back from New York, she stopped in Philadelphia where she and her husband grew up. They went to visit a family she had become close to. Out of high school, Desi was a nanny for a year or so. Her best friend also became a nanny. In the best friend's family were two attorneys. One day, the wife had been doing sidewalk counseling outside an abortion clinic. The lady she was talking to told her that if she would adopt the baby, she would not go through with the abortion. The attorney mentioned she was an attorney and would write up the papers personally.

She and her husband adopted this little boy. When he started school, they recognized that he had some significant difficulties in learning to read. Somewhere in his early grades, they discovered he was a child prodigy for piano playing. He could not read the music, but he could hear it and play it.

He had two music teachers, one from Russia who did not care that he could not read the music because he knew he felt it. The other music teacher was a little bit frustrated because she could not help him with reading the music. He would see the music one note at a time just the way he would read one word at a time.

Desi, my vision therapist, was hearing this story and thought, "Why don't you try these glasses on?" She pulled out her lovely women's Silhouette frames and had the young man, who was eleven or twelve years old, put them on. It instantly tripled his reading speed. She left the glasses with him to use until he could get in to see a colleague of mine whom I contacted and explained how to do the testing for the lens. He took the glasses to his piano lesson. As they opened the score, he could read the music and play.

This story still absolutely amazes me. How so many events came together at just the right time in just the right sequence. Thankfully, my rudeness was also part of the plan. Diane did not need light therapy, which was the reason I had called in the first place years before. It was perfect timing for meeting Dr. Collier over the phone and then coordinating his visit to Spokane. It was perfect for whose name was pulled out of the hat. GOD is good!

Diane's story was our introduction to this very special lens.

BINARY LENSES 2

It is all about timing. Think of the prisms we had in grade school that would turn white light into a rainbow of colors. That occurs because it is bending the light in different amounts to create the different colors or wavelengths. Another way of saying prisms change by bending light is that they are changing the phase or timing of light.

In our brain stem or midbrain, there are incredible connections where eye movements, auditory (hearing), vestibular (inner ear balance), and body awareness (proprioception) all connect and feed back to one another. These senses create a "clearer picture" of where we are in space and where different parts of our body are positioned. Some major proprioception receptors are found in the ankles, knees, hips, neck, and finger joints. These give awareness of various body part's position, movement, and awareness of gravity.

The top part of the brainstem is called the superior colliculus. Seventy percent of the nerves in the superior colliculus are connected with the eyes, but these nerves have nothing to do with eyesight. But the connections do have a lot to do regarding timing. The nerves involved with sight travel at 60-70 milliseconds (thousandths of a second). But, the non-sight nerves in the brainstem travel at 15-20 milliseconds as do the hearing, balance, and body awareness nerves. So the non-sight nerves are about four times faster than nerves used for sight!

The yoked prism lenses change the timing of light to the midbrain, and the body can respond to extremely minute amounts of differences to cause change. This would be described in a number of examples of patients we have worked with since meeting Dr. Collier in 2003.

One patient in her early forties was the wife of a general physician in town. She had had some health issues all throughout her life. As her husband said, Western medicine does not have all the answers. They had gone every-where and done everything traditionally, and no one could figure out why she had issues with thinking clearly as well as walking. She was using crutches with braces on the forearm to move around and had been since she was in high school.

She came back for a further performance evaluation. Part of that involved testing her for the yoked prisms. My vision therapists do the evaluation, and when she was seated in the exam room after the testing, I saw that the chart had "Wow!!!!!!" under the yoked prism testing.

Initially when we had asked her to walk a line on the floor forward and backward, even with her crutches, she could not get her foot to land on the line despite numerous attempts. Then the therapist tried different orienta-tions of the yoked prisms. With the first pair, there was no response. With the second pair, there was no response. With the third pair the patient put on, she paused, looked around, let go of her crutches, and walked unaided heel to toe both forward and backward along the line on the floor. She started to cry, then her husband started to cry as they were hugging each other.

With the three of us in the exam room, her husband started shaking his head in disbelief. His wife was looking around the room with the glasses on and said, "Do you mean I don't have to feel like I'm drunk all the time?"

Her husband said, "Let me see this again. I just have to see this. Let me take the glasses." She handed them to him, and he asked her to stand up. With great wobbling and difficulty, she was able to stand up but still needed to hold on to the arm of the examination chair for stability. Then she sat back down. He then handed her the glasses. She put them on. Without hesitation, she quickly stood up without having to hold on to anything. She sat down. He was shaking his head in disbelief.

I said, "You haven't seen anything yet. Let me have the glasses. Close your eyes. Please stand up." She attempted. She wobbled and wobbled. She could not stand up with her eyes closed. I then had her put the glasses on. "Close your eyes. Stand up." Immediately, without hesitation, she was able to stand with her eyes closed without holding on to anything. This really got their attention. Since the brainstem has nothing to do with sight itself, and there is still light going through closed eyelids, it was further a demonstration that the prism changes the timing of light to the brain.

Another story is about a sixty-nine-year-old gentleman from the Seattle area whom we saw a few years back. He initially heard about our office from his niece who had come to us while she was attempting to go to college but had to drop out because of poor grades and an inability to comprehend what she was reading. In her case, she immediately benefited from the prism lenses and then began to do syntonic or light therapy to allow her to use a greater amount of information at a time. Between the two, she was able to signifi-cantly improve her eye coordination, go back to college, get on the honor roll, and graduate.

When her uncle heard about her trials and then success, he was definitely interested. At age sixty-nine, he had throughout his entire schooling and adult life only been able to read ten minutes at a time before he would have to stop. It was useless to continue reading because his comprehension was so poor due to the agonizingly slow reading speed.

He came in for an examination, and we found he had a very difficult time converging or making his eyes aim inward for reading. He showed a significant improvement instantly with the yoked prism lenses. He also had a reduced near-point functional vision field and would benefit from the syntonic light therapy.

During the case history, it turned out he had throughout his life had major issues with anxiety and actually learned hypnosis to help him when he was out in public. If there were too many people around him, he learned how he could somewhat calm his system through self-hypnosis in order to deal with the increased stimulation from the environment.

We gave him a prescription for the prism lenses. He went home to Seattle, filled the prescription, and did the light therapy. When we saw him six weeks later, his near-point functional field had completely opened, and he reported that he was thoroughly enjoying reading for the first time in his life. He was reading two to three hours at a time each day, happily devouring books because he could read much faster and comprehend what he was reading.

When I asked him about his anxiety, he paused and thought. He realized, "Wow. That is considerably better." In fact, something had happened the week before. Normally, it would have totally caused a panic attack, but he realized he just dealt with the issue, moved on, and did not give it a second thought.

Another wonderful story was with a ten-year-old girl with cerebral palsy who had been working in physical therapy for two to three years to try to help her walk smoothly and in balance. She also had been using the forearm brace crutches to help her maintain her balance. With the prism lens in place, she was able to instantly put down the crutches and walk forward and backward unaided for the first time that her mother had ever seen.

The prism lens is not a cure-all for all people with balance issues, but it certainly warrants a trial to see if it can be of assistance.

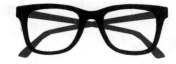

TRAUMATIC BRAIN INJURY

Imagine you are driving in a parking lot looking for a space to pull in. You see something off to your right side, and all of a sudden there is a jarring, and you hear a crunch when you realize someone has just backed into your car.

It is a horrible feeling just thinking of the hassle that is involved. What if later in the day you feel a little funny, and you brush it off due to the stress of the accident? What if four to eight weeks later, your frustration level is slowly increasing, and it seems like you are having a harder time concentrating? What if your ability to comprehend and read seems to become more difficult? You think, "Am I getting old? Is it my glasses that are off? It might be stress." You notice that your loved one is annoying you more, and you just like to be left alone. Then you think, "I wonder if I'm depressed." You go see your family physician who listens to this and writes a prescription for an antidepressant.

Slowly, gradually, your life is changed. Could it have been from that fender-bender in the parking lot several months before?

As we find out later in this chapter, there is story upon story of examples of patients I have seen who have had changes in their lives from traumatic brain injury which influenced the visual system's ability to process information. It can be an extremely subtle condition. Those with traumatic brain injury are known as the "walking wounded" because from outward appearance, they look totally fine. Even looking at them with a number of diagnostic instruments, from CAT scans to MRI, everything looks completely fine. "It must be in their head," doctors often say.

In this chapter, we will be discussing traumatic brain injury related to difficulties in the individual system and how often therapies can be done that can make a profound impact in regaining improved quality of life so you can enjoy life again. Depending on the severity of the trauma, things may not go back to the way they used to be. However, before resigning oneself to a much lower quality of life, a person should have their visual system evaluated in a way that looks at the function and more than just whether the pathway from the eyeball to the brain is intact and healthy.

The visual system has five times the sensory input to the brain of any other sense in our body. Approximately 25 percent of our total energy consumption daily is used by the visual system. This has very little to do with our ability to see clearly but more with how our eyes coordinate. In particular, how do we process the information coming in through the eyes? This is the area that can be significantly impacted by head trauma.

Let's go back to the parking lot fender-bender. It was subtle. It did not cause the airbags to deploy. There was minimal damage to the bumper. Could something little like that cause a problem? Think of the anatomy of our body. Our head weighs approximately eleven to twelve pounds. It is on our neck, so depending on the length of our neck, the robustness of the muscles that support our neck, and our body structure, different impacts can have different amounts of damage. A ninety-five-pound person will not be able to sustain the same amount of impact that a three-hundred-pound linebacker would be able to sustain.

Imagine a bullwhip. As you take the handle into your hand and make that snap movement, the speed of the end of the whip is going so fast that it breaks the sound barrier. It is that amount of whipping motion that can cause difficulties. A five-mile-an-hour parking lot fender-bender can put five thousand pounds of force on a person's brain stem. A thirty-mile-an-hour accident can easily put over thirty thousand pounds of force on the brain stem.

We have all hit our funny bone and noted that unpleasant feeling when it is hit. We start shaking it off because of that pain. That is a sudden impact on a nerve in the elbow. Imagine our brain stem getting a sudden jolt or impact from the whipping motion caused by the impact.

You can have a similar type of physiological reaction as hitting your funny bone, but have it happening to your brain stem, and it is not so funny. I do not want to dive too deeply into the physiology, but know that there are neurotransmitters involved. Those are the chemicals that help run our brain and nervous system. Calcium and potassium are part of the nerve signaling. If there is a sudden impact, just like when you hit your funny bone, those nerves are now activated, and that "uses" up a molecule.

Along with this sudden impact or depolarization of the nerve, there is a void. Nature abhors a vacuum, so calcium, which is part of every cell, will rush in to balance out this polarization. However, the unfortunate part of it is that too much calcium can be toxic to nerves. This "calcium cascade" can lead to issues surfacing weeks, even months, after the initial injury. Feel free to google "calcium cascade related to traumatic brain injury" or "neurometabolic cascade of concussion." The consequences of this calcium cascade can be incredibly detrimental.

Clark Elliott, a DePaul University professor in artificial intelligence, wrote a book in 2015 called *The Ghost in my Brain*. It is a wonderful book by a person with firsthand experience to traumatic brain injury and the years it took for him to deal with it and ultimately receive some incredible therapy to help him regain his life. He is most grateful to Deborah Zelinsky, a doctor of optometry, in the Chicago area for being of such tremendous assistance to him.

Along with the physiological changes that go along with a traumatic brain injury, how a person experiences it in their day-to-day life is what is most important to them. A common theme throughout this book is looking at different parts of the nervous system related to the visual system under duress or stress, whether it is a traumatic brain injury, stroke, or a child who had a traumatic birth, or even while in utero the mother was under severe trauma. All these varied amounts of physical or emotional stress have similar impact on our body's nervous system.

In a review of the syntonics chapter about the sympathetic and parasympathetic nervous system, you will see those very common symptoms found in traumatic brain injury. These can include photophobia, or light sensitivity, increased sensitivity to other inputs, whether it is sound or texture, or movement can be particularly bothersome. It is not uncommon for a person to start having digestive difficulties following a traumatic brain injury due to the decrease in stomach acid caused by the sympathetic dominant nervous system. Balance or ease with walking can be affected by the traumatic brain injury. Short-term memory and sleep issues are also not uncommon. The symptoms go on and on as to how injury to the head or neck can have quite a significant impact on a person's life.

One example is a patient who was a physical therapist until eight years prior. He slipped on ice and hit the back of his head. At that point forward until this day, he has been unable to work due to the consequence of events over the next several months that unfolded before his eyes. He was having greater difficulty doing his physical therapy work and being able to concentrate on what he was doing. Since then, he has been on a search for ways to get better.

He was referred to our office from another doctor who had been working with him on some vision therapies that were helping him develop improved skills. However, there were still some pieces missing. When we saw the gentleman, it was found that the binary or yoked prism lenses instantly had an impact on improving his reading fluency and speed. We found that the syntonic light therapy proved to be very helpful for him, as well as a method of increasing microcirculation, which you will find in another chapter in this book. He lives three hours away from our office, and his ability to ride home was much more comfortable when he received the benefit of increased circulation as well as a nudge into the balancing of his nervous systems.

Strokes are another type of traumatic brain injury with the loss of blood flow to certain parts of the brain. Classically, when eye doctors think of the visual system in strokes, we think of people who may have a homonymous hemianopsia. That is a tongue-twisting way of saying the person is unable to see either the right or left side of their visual field. This type of vision loss is incredibly debilitating. The worse of the two is when it is the right field that is no longer intact. When we read English, we read from the left to the right, so if the ability to scan to the right does not provide any visual information, reading speed and accuracy are significantly impaired.

That brings us to one simple technique that can be extremely helpful for someone with right visual field loss. There is nothing cast in stone saying we have to hold our book in the manner in which we usually do. If a person with a right field loss turned their book ninety degrees clockwise, the text would now be running top to bottom and flowing from right to left so that a person would be moving in the direction of their usable peripheral vision.

Homonymous Hemianopsia

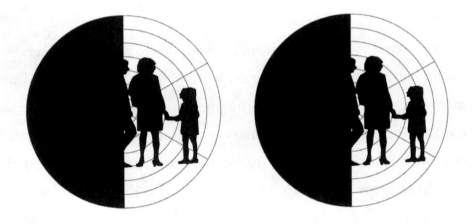

This is not something that is beneficial immediately, but if a person is willing to practice changing the way they do things, they could start to learn to move their eyes from top to bottom, and then move to the left reading top to bottom using the remaining visual field they have. They have to be willing to practice. It is somewhat like learning to read again. However, it is interesting how quickly a person can start to pick up the ability to read vertically or even when the text is upside down.

The vast majority of patients I have seen who have had strokes do not have this half-vision loss in each eye, but they do have varying amounts of functional visual field loss. This relates to the syntonics chapter. Doctors who are involved with the syntonic light therapy typically measure functional visual fields with a moving target, not just using "Push the button. Did you see the light or did you not?" testing devices.

The movement visual field provides a great deal more information related to a person's visual function and higher levels of brain processing. Essentially, how much change can take place in a person's peripheral vision before they notice there is a change, first with movement, and then are they able to discern a change in color? These are all very helpful in formulating a therapy plan to try to maximize the recovery for the patient.

This was very clearly seen in two patients who come to mind. One patient in her seventies came into the office accompanied by her husband pushing her in her wheelchair. She had had a stroke, and one of the main symptoms was that while she loved reading before the stroke, she found reading extremely frustrating and very tiresome. Her husband noted that she was also quite frustrated in day-to-day life, and little things that used to be of no concern were quite concerning for her. She overall had considerable anxiety throughout the day.

We found that she was still able to see clearly out of each eye. However, she did have significant difficulty with eye tracking skills as well as her ability to make her eyes work as a team during reading. We measured her near-point functional visual field (see the syntonics chapter) and she had considerable tunneling of her near-point peripheral vision in each eye.

Functional Tunnel Vision

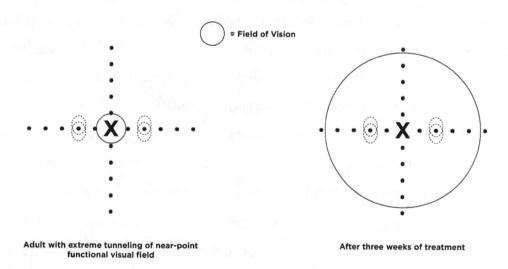

○ = Field of Vision

Adult with extreme tunneling of near-point
functional visual field

After three weeks of treatment

One other issue apparent with this lady's situation is quite common with head trauma patients as well as stroke patients. Prior to the injury, they may have done quite well with progressive or no-line bifocals. The no-line progressive has a corridor where, as a person looks down, it gradually increases the power in the lens, so objects at intermediate as well as reading distance are in focus. There is a narrow channel which the eyes need to track through and maintain alignment to use this lens properly. When someone has had an injury and loses some of the coordination and control of his eyes, the progressive lens can become more difficult to use and be another source of frustration. That was the case with this patient, so we wrote a prescription for her to have a pair of glasses for distance vision and a separate one just for reading. She also was given syntonic light therapy to work on helping open up her peripheral awareness.

We saw her a few weeks later, and her countenance was considerably improved. The sparkle was back in her eye. She mentioned she was thoroughly enjoying reading once again and was no longer in need of the wheelchair because her balance had improved as well.

We saw this in another gentleman in his late eighties who was a rancher from a town a couple of hours south of Spokane, Washington. He still had been riding horses and watching over things on his ranch, and then he likely had a mild stroke. The doctors were unable to pinpoint it exactly, but he noticed a considerable decrease in his reading ability as well. Just like the previous lady, his ability to read had become much more difficult. He was no longer enjoying it and was very frustrated. His near-point peripheral awareness visual field test showed considerable tunneling of peripheral vision.

He greatly benefited from the balancing of the sympathetic and parasympathetic nervous system, which helped open up his peripheral awareness and allowed him to read much more easily. When the peripheral vision is tunneled, a person is unable to efficiently use his peripheral vision to know where to move his eyes when he is reading. We "feed forward" using our peripheral vision, which actually starts preprocessing the reading and narrows down what words are likely coming so that by the time our eyes are directed onto those words, we have already a pretty good idea of what the words are. If someone is unable to access that peripheral awareness, it greatly impedes reading speed because the preprocessing is not able to be accessed, and that slows the reading, increases the effort spent, and increases fatigue.

As you read about the patients, whether it is with traumatic brain injury, suffering from anxiety, or others with vision-related learning disabilities, you will see a common theme of visual symptoms as well as other day-to-day life experiences that are negatively impacted from poor coordination or an inefficiently operating visual system. The good news is that in the vast majority of cases, things can be done to help ease the effort spent and assist with improving performance. We certainly cannot guarantee anything for any patient, but the brain is amazingly pliable and retrainable. It is always worthwhile to look into the different options for helping patients gain improved quality of life.

NUTRITION AND VISION

"I'm eating carrots, so my eyes should be fine." While carrots are okay for your eyes and your general health, it is much more complex than just eating carrots. In this chapter, we will be discussing reasons why a person should pay close attention to their nutrition if they want their visual system working at an optimal level.

Here is some eye trivia. The retina, the back of the eye that receives light information, has the highest metabolic need of any tissue in our body. The retina is literally a sea of blood vessels with an incredibly vast complex network of tiny capillaries providing nutrients, oxygen, and waste removal for the millions of light receptors.

Jerry Tennant, MD, is one of the preeminent eye surgeons in the United States (www.TennantInstitute.us). He notes that the macula, the pinpoint of sharpest sight in the eye, is turning over cells every two days because of the incredible metabolic demand of the part of our retina which gives us the clear sight for reading and driving.

The eyes are processing eighteen billion data bits per second between the two retinas. It is not too much of a stretch to realize that what we take into our bodies day after day will have a significant impact on the health of various organs, and the eye is certainly no exception.

In my opinion, the eyes can certainly be a canary in the coal mine. Early changes in the macular condition or macular function can be precursors to what is happening throughout the rest of the body and can reflect overall health. Due to this high metabolic demand of the retina, it is also why, in a number of patients, we can see quite rapid changes in improvement in their visual system, because it is so metabolically sensitive.

One eighty-three-year-old patient we saw in the office in July 2013 was visiting his daughter for two weeks in Spokane as he lives in Baja, Mexico, because he loves to fish. He has a history of dry macular degeneration. His best corrected acuity was 20/40 in his good eye. This is the minimum needed for an unrestricted driver's license. His worse eye was 20/70. Because he was in town for such a short time, we had him start the comprehensive nutrient supplement by Biosyntrx (Eye and Body formula) as well as purpose to drink one to two ounces of filtered water every thirty minutes that he was awake. He also began in-office sessions with a device that helps blood flow through-out the whole body. He did this session eight minutes a day for eight days out of ten, and he was able to demonstrate a two-line improvement in vision in each eye.

We had also done a baseline measurement with a visual evoked potential. This is a device where we place electrodes onto his scalp, and it records the timing of light from the instant it hits the retina. It measures how long it takes for it to reach the back of the brain, which is the occipital cortex, or vision center of the brain. It is measured in milliseconds, and a three-millisecond change is significant. His good eye sped up by nine milliseconds and his worse eye by just under six milliseconds.

Needless to say, he and his daughter were extremely pleased, and he has continued to benefit from the nutrients as well as the increased circulation from the device. As of July 2016, for the first time, he was able to read one letter on the 20/20 line in his good eye. At age eighty-six, his quality of life had some other significant benefits as well. Within that year in 2013, he was able to start riding a bicycle. He also bought a Kindle and has been happily enjoying ebooks ever since.

As seen throughout this book, the importance of circulation to the retina is crucial, as it is to our whole body. Chronic stress has a significant detrimental effect on the body's ability to circulate blood and get the nutrients to where they need to go. Anything that can be done to help with that blood flow is extremely important. The quality of the blood, as far as what nutrients are able to be transporting to the cells, is hugely significant. Unfortunately, with the SAD, Standard American Diet, nutrient quality has continued to decline year after year.

The eyes and brain are 50 percent fat, so to have someone mention you are a fathead is a compliment! The quality of the fats we eat is extremely important. Much has been written on the deleterious effects of hydrogenated fats in our diet. That is certainly true with the visual system as well. Good quality fats as well as the body's ability to assimilate those fats is extremely important. If someone has digestive difficulties or is missing a gallbladder, it becomes much more difficult for the body to assimilate the fats, break them down into components that can be used by the body, and get them to the different parts of the eye and nervous system to help them function.

Sources of good-quality fats would include Alaska wild salmon and avocados. A couple of other sources that are not as widely known are hemp hearts and chia seeds as well as a new source I learned of this summer at a farmers' market here in Spokane called camelina oil (www.CamelinaGold. com).

One source of camelina is grown sixty miles away from Spokane in Ritzville, Washington. It really is remarkable oil. It is a 35 percent plant-based omega-3 oil. It has a 475-degree smoke point, so it is extremely stable for cooking. Please look into that as a helpful source for your body for obtaining a very good quality oil. This can also be helpful for people with dry eye situations as well as with dry skin. (Interestingly, the Navy used camelina as a source for some biofuel studies…I hate to imagine what the cost of the biofuel was per gallon, but that is a different story.)

Continued research is being done on the pigments in the macula and how they are helpful in protecting the macula from ultraviolet damage from light as well as possible damage from the blue end of the visible light spectrum. Zeaxanthin and lutein are a couple of the pigments that appear to be helpful in reducing the potential for macular damage. There are instruments now available for measuring macular pigment optical density. It is a measurement that can be helpful in monitoring a person's ability to resist damage from those sources of light.

Kale is the king of foods for lutein concentration. It has approximately twenty-six times the amount of lutein as spinach. Red peppers are a great source of zeaxanthin. If a person wants to make some kale chips and put some hot sauce on them, it is a nice one-two combo for getting both macular pigments into the body. If a person is not a kale fan, supplements can be taken. In the office, we are able to measure the improvements in macular pigment optical density that can take place over a six-month period of time when a person is taking a good quality zeaxanthin and lutein supplement with meals.

A person's digestive system is crucial. A well-working system is extremely helpful, as we have had a few patients who have compromised digestive systems. Their ability to assimilate zeaxanthin and lutein is significantly slower or impaired due to their poor digestive abilities.

Another supplement that has been helpful for the eyes and brain is astaxanthin. It sounds like it should be a cousin of zeaxanthin, but it is not that close of a cousin. You can read more about the benefits of astaxanthin on Dr. Joseph Mercola's website (www.Mercola.com). It helps with oxygen intake to the brain and eyes and has the nice side benefit of appearing to help decrease the chance of getting sunburn due to the pigment that is in the astaxanthin.

Anecdotally, I had a gastroenterologist as a patient who was beginning to notice a slight decrease in distance acuity and the very slight beginnings of cataracts. He had not been a big supporter of nutritional supplements, but I mentioned that he might want to consider giving them a try.

He was pleasantly surprised to report two weeks later that he noticed a significant improvement in clarity. He enjoyed target practice with a pistol. He had had difficulty with sight acquisition, and he was amazed that he was able to now see both the front and back sight of his pistol after just two weeks of using the astaxanthin. It had been a couple of years since he had been able to have that same vision. Needless to say, he has been a continued fan of astaxanthin for his ocular health.

I would highly recommend people increase their education on the significance of our gut flora as that relates to our overall health. A book written in 2015 by neurologist David Perlmutter, MD, called *Brain Maker: The Power of Gut Microbes to Heal and Protect* is a very timely and informative book pointing out current research going on with our gut flora and the incredible impact it has on our health. As he notes, certain bacteria are responsible for gene expression, so it is absolutely essential that people become more familiar with what they can do to enhance their gut flora and minimize damage to the ten trillion friendlies in a healthy person's digestion tract.

I recommend people also become more aware of the many benefits of naturally fermented foods. Naturally fermented sauerkraut can have 316 billion probiotic colonies per teaspoon. Our entire gut flora is about ten trillion probiotic colonies, so a tablespoon of sauerkraut would provide almost one trillion good bacteria. A number of patients with digestive difficulties have been extremely pleased with how much their digestive ability has improved once they started consuming the naturally fermented foods.

I would like to take a little side tour and talk about light. You might be asking, "Is light related to nutrition?" Bear with me. I will let you decide if it is a possibility.

The research on the biological effects of light has continued to explode over the last ten to fifteen years. If you want a quick glimpse, google "LLLT, low level light therapy, eye and brain" for an article by Dove Press reviewing a great number of studies related to the biological effects of light.

At the 2014 Syntonic Light Therapy Conference in Saint Pete's Beach, Florida, James Oschman, PhD, biophysicist from Delaware, was talking about some of the recent discoveries by biophysicists related to light. He said they have realized that each photon (the smallest particle of light man has defined) is capable of carrying not just one piece of data but also a string of data. That alone is worthy of a pause to reflect on what that means.

As this book is being written, commercial application of that discovery is taking place. By the time this book is published in the next few months, the term LiFi will become more of a household word. We are all familiar with WiFi. This is LiFi, referring to light. This will be well over one hundred times faster than WiFi for download because of the ability to attach strings of data for each photon. Presently, they are able to download the equivalent of forty-seven single sided DVDs in one second using light as the medium. I am sure one of the next iPhones will likely have the capability of receiving this light signal for data downloading.

There will be some limitations since it is line of sight. It will also have some advantages for security purposes. They will be able to put a microchip in an LED light bulb and a light sensor on the computer or cell phone. If the light is on, the internet connection is activated for transfer of data.

It is well established that light is an incredible carrier of information. What about a biophoton or a life-produced particle of light? In the book, *Biophotons —The Lights in our Cells*, Marco Bischof notes, "According to the biophoton theory developed on the base of these discoveries, the biophoton light is stored in the cells of the organism—more precisely, in the DNA molecules of their nuclei—and a dynamic web of light constantly released and absorbed by the DNA may connect cell organelles, cells, tissues, and organs within the body and serve as the organism's main communication network and as the principal regulating instance for all life processes." Please take a moment to reread and reflect on that paragraph. Ponder the huge significance of biophotons in the operation of every cell in our body.

Back to the discussion on nutrition, when we think of vine-ripened fruits and vegetables, the pigments or flavonoids in the fruit or vegetable are maximized when the fruit or vegetable is ripe. What are the possibilities that there is an incredible amount of data contained in the biophotons or life-produced particles of light in vine-ripened fruits or vegetables that was designed for our benefit, yet we have no clue of what all is contained in those biophotons? Also consider what are the quality and quantity of biophotons available in vine-ripened fruits and vegetables compared to, if there is even such a thing, a biophoton or life-produced particle of light in a chicken nugget from a fast food restaurant? That's literally "food for thought."

If these biophotons are most prevalent in vine-ripened fruits and vegetables, how often are we able to buy vine-ripened fruits and vegetables? Depending on where a person lives in the country, they may be accessible from a local farmer's market a good part of the year, or it may be just a very short window of opportunity to buy locally grown produce that you can get when it is at its peak ripeness.

What if there was a product available where seventy to eighty pounds of vine-ripened fruits and vegetables were very low heat dehydrated to keep the enzymes viable? What if all the oxygen, almost all the water, and 98 percent of the sugar was removed and condensed down so those seventy to eighty pounds ended up fitting in an eight-and-a-half-ounce jar? What if a quarter-teaspoon serving size of this product was the equivalent of consuming the nutrients from one and one half to two pounds of fruits and vegetables? What if the product was put in the mouth, and as you let it linger and rolled it around in the mouth, a good percentage of the nutrients were transferred sublingually without having to go through a digestive system that may or may not be working efficiently?

I recommend that you do due diligence and look into Flavon products from Hungary. They are distributed in the United States from Flavon USA in Florida. It is one of the easiest ways a person can have available to them high quality nutrients from fruits and vegetables year round. Please see my website for further details.

The discussion on nutrition would not be complete without bringing up the topic of toxins and the detrimental effect they have on our body functions. I greatly appreciate Dr. Tennant's insight into the many sources of toxins into our body from things we eat but also different exposures we have with modified foods to potential impact of dental infections. If you have any chronic health problems, I would highly recommend you look at his website for further discussion in this area.

A few years ago, a fifty-two-year-old patient came to my office wanting a second opinion on her glaucoma. Glaucoma is an eye condition where the optic nerve starts to lose function, in many cases related to eye pressure. However, 50 percent of glaucoma patients have normal eye pressure, so it is not strictly related to pressure in the eye. Recently, there has been the discussion on whether glaucoma is really more of a brain disease. This fits with the metabolic approach to eye health. If there is interference with oxygen, nutrients, or waste removal going on in the optic nerve, that seems to be a reasonable explanation for why a person's nerve could begin to show damage, the effect of which appears to be glaucoma.

This patient had "normal" eye pressure but also pretty extensive damage demonstrated in the thickness of her optic nerve fiber layer. This can be measured with an ocular coherence tomography (OCT). There are norms for the population of thickness. Listening to the patient's case history, it became apparent that she had a number of other health issues with digestion and extensive dental history with a high number of amalgam fillings. I am aware that the American Dental Association says there is no health problem with the amalgam fillings, which contain mercury. It is interesting to note that while that filling that contains mercury is "safe" in our mouth, if that same amount of mercury is placed into a pond, from the Environmental Protection Agency's point of view, it is deemed a hazard to health.

I referred the patient to a naturopath, and they were able to find that she had very high mercury content. She did some heavy metal detoxing and was able to observe, over the next several months, an improvement in her optic nerve layer thickness as measured by the OCT.

She came in this past year, and the nerve fiber layer was starting to thin again despite the detoxing. This is anecdotal, but she did have one crown left. She went to a dentist and asked to have that tooth removed. The dentist was hesitant because it appeared that the tooth was sound, but at the patient's request, he went ahead. As he took the top of the crown off, he was amazed to see a large amount of amalgam filling that had been capped over. Once the tooth was removed, the patient came back into the office. Once again, we are seeing the nerve fiber layer starting to increase in thickness. Coincidence? Maybe.

In conclusion, the importance of nutrients for the eye cannot be underestimated. Please use the aforementioned resources to help your eyes and your body benefit from improving the availability of good quality nutrients. You will not be sorry.

VISUAL HYGIENE

No, this is not a chapter on ways to keep your eyes clean and sanitary. It is looking at ways to help your visual system be more efficient and decrease the possibilities of your children ending up with nearsightedness or astigmatism.

Our world's increasing dependence upon iPhones, iPads, and computers has definitely taken a toll on our visual health. These objects are not necessarily physiologically impairing our health, but the function, flexibility, and comfort of using our eyes can be compromised by these devices.

Our eye is the only organ in the body that has two different nervous systems operating different parts of it at the same time. Movement through space helps the development and coordination of these two nervous systems. A child learns to gain better motor control over his different body parts by moving through space guided by the visual system. I cannot emphasize more strongly the need for children to play, move, and do three-dimensional real-world activities. It is so easy to use flat screens as babysitters, but they are not helping children's vision development or visual motor skills.

Please significantly limit the amount of time they spend using the tablet devices to help their development. We are in a three-dimensional world, but those objects are two-dimensional. It is becoming more and more of a problem as we are seeing children who do not know how to efficiently move their bodies through space.

The other part that is so easy to do is to allow extended periods of time using the tablet and iPhones. It is so easy to get sucked into those devices, and time flies by. Studies have been done showing that as we engage with these devices, our respiration and blink rate slow down. We become so engaged that basic metabolic functions start to slow.

It is so important from an early age to teach children to spend a maximum of fifteen or twenty minutes doing sustained near-point work and then take a break. Spend at least a minute or so moving, getting a drink of water, looking out a window, and moving and breathing to help refresh the eye.

As adults, the same thing applies. We will be far more efficient when we are doing computer work if we take breaks every twenty minutes and allow our visual system to "refresh." For students of any age, please look at my "Study Smarter, Not Harder" report giving a number of study tips to make studying easier, almost fun, and definitely more productive.

Another part of visual hygiene relates to the type of light coming off our computer devices. The blue-white light is a daytime color. There have been at least two studies related to iPad users using them for two hours in the evening. After two hours of use over a two-month period of time, melatonin production dropped 11 percent. This is extremely important for getting good-quality sleep. More and more people are having difficulty getting a good night's rest because of the exposure to the concentrated daytime light color temperature coming off our devices.

Please look into downloading free software, which can be very helpful for decreasing this problem. It is well worth looking into www.JustGetFlux.com or www.IrisTech.co. Both apps will automatically warm the color temperature of your device in the evening hours, which significantly decreases the interference with our circadian rhythm.

As mentioned, if we get in the habit of locking in for near-point work, our respiration and blink rate decrease. I had a patient a number of years ago who was the epitome of this situation. This patient was in her mid-forties and was a medical doctor on disability due to severe digestive issues. She was an extremely kind person but had a Type A personality off the scale. She was a very intense person wound like a clock, as they say.

She had one of the most severe cases of dry eye that I had ever heard. She had been to ten ophthalmologists in ten years seeking any sort of assistance. Her eyes constantly ached every waking moment. She had punctal plugs put in her eyelids to decrease the amount of fluid draining from the eye. She had used every dry eye product on the market.

Her "solution" for survival was to use eye drops extensively during the day, and then at night she would put a blob of Lacri-Lube, a very thick ointment for severe dry eyes somewhat the consistency of toothpaste, in each eye. She would then wrap her eye area with Saran Wrap™ to make a moisture chamber to keep the moisture from the Lacri-Lube in her eyes. Then she would use a thick two-inch hair band to keep the Saran Wrap™ in place. This mental picture does create an interesting look. That had been her mode of survival to deal with the agony of her dry eyes.

I look back at this as one of the God moments in my career. I felt prompted to ask her to consider reading the book *Relearning to See* by Tom Quackenbush. Because of her off-the-charts Type A personality, it seemed appropriate to suggest she take a new look at how she could use her eyes.

I loaned her my copy of the book and did not think anything else about it until two months later when she stopped by the office, and she was on cloud nine! She asked to see me, and as I entered the exam room, she started saying, "Thank you so very much for helping me." I was taken aback a little bit and thought, "What did I do?"

She mentioned how she had started to read *Relearning to See* and read the chapter on blinking. She realized that with her intense personality, she had overridden and totally deactivated her normal blink reflex. Throughout the day, she was just staring at everything and almost never blinking. She did the blinking exercises mentioned in the book, and in two weeks, all her dry eye symptoms had totally vanished!

She was beside herself with joy because now she could read again for pleasure. She had been unable to do so for several years. Within a few months, she was able to write an article on gut bacteria, which was accepted for publication by a medical journal. She was kind enough to give an acknowledgment in the foreword to her article thanking me for assisting in her recovery from her severe dry eyes. That story, to me, is the height of the simplest of cures for a severe problem.

One line of dry eye product that we have found very helpful for dry eye treatment is a product from Natural Ophthalmics, a homeopathic company out of Colorado. Their gel drop, which can be used at nighttime, has been very effective for a number of patients.

Most of the repair of our corneal cells takes place at night, and we turn over a new corneal epithelium—top layer of the cornea—every seven to ten days. There are extreme metabolic changes taking place at the corneal level as well. When a person has a tendency toward dry eye and his new cells are getting laid down and repaired at night, if some of those cells end up sticking to the inside of the eyelid, it is going to peel off just like a Band-Aid pulling a scab when the person wakes in the morning. It can pull off some of those newly formed cells causing a recurrence of the injury to the cornea. It can set up for a recurrent corneal abrasion or erosion where night after night the repair continues to be peeled back.

The Natural Ophthalmics gel drop has been very effective for helping not only to provide increased thickness of moisture and decrease the possibility of the cells being removed, but the homeopathic properties in the drops are tending to nudge the body in the direction of helping fix the underlying problem leading to the dry eye. Please see my website for the availability of these drops.

Another area related to dry eye that has profoundly greater significance for general health is the use of artificial sweeteners. I have had several patients over the years where we have seen a significant dry eye and eye discomfort associated with the use of artificial sweeteners.

One of the first instances was several years ago when we were fitting a fifteen-year-old young man with soft contact lenses. Several months before, we had fit one of his older sisters with soft contacts, so when he came in to get contact lenses, I did a diagnostic fitting using the same brand of lenses that his sister was successfully using. We put on the lenses and let them settle for fifteen minutes. When we went to check his vision, surprisingly, he could not see the 20/20 line in each eye, and vision was blurry. There was no additional lens power I could place over the top of the contact lenses that improved acuity.

When I looked with the microscope at his eyes, the contact lenses literally had a coating. It looked like the lenses of someone who had over worn their contacts and had not taken them out for weeks. There was a mucous film on the contacts definitely accounting for the decreased acuity. This was in a fifteen-year-old "healthy" young man.

In questioning him, I happened to ask if he was hydrating. He said he was drinking water. I asked about any other fluids he was drinking. He said, "I have a diet pop in my lunch that I take to school every day." Knowing there are a number of articles related to harmful effects associated with artificial sweeteners, I asked him to run a science experiment. For the next three weeks, he stopped taking the diet pop with him to school and drank water instead.

We saw him three weeks later and tried the exact same type of contact lens in his eyes. After letting the contacts settle, fifteen minutes later he could clearly read better than 20/20 in each eye. The contacts were wetting perfectly, and there was no sign of the film that we had seen three weeks prior. This has continued to be not an uncommon occurrence in our office with contact lens wearers who are having, for unknown reasons, issues with contact lens comfort or clarity.

I had one patient with MS who was having dry eyes and had been using a walker for a number of years because of the difficulty of her balance related to the MS. I mentioned that she should run this science experiment and stop using artificial sweeteners to see what happens. It turns out I was the second of three people in the same day who suggested she do the same thing for various reasons, so she ended up discontinuing use of the artificial sweetener. One week later, she found she no longer needed her walker to assist her in walking.

Though the artificial sweeteners are approved by the FDA, I would highly recommend anyone using them to reconsider and look into the many studies that show they do not help with weight loss but are often associated with significant other health difficulties.

LIFE IS IN THE BLOOD

Life is in the blood. We know that if our heart stops, our moments of life are quickly numbered. What we will take a look at in this chapter is not only the impact of blood flow for the whole body but also regarding how it influences the effect of our precious gift of sight. What if there is something you can do to help your blood flow and it does not involve exercise? We will be discussing that in this chapter.

To take a look at how blood flows in our capillaries and to see the effect chronic stress has on our capillary blood flow, I would urge you to go to the website of Rainer Klopp, MD, from Berlin, Germany. He is the medical director for the Institute for Microcirculation in Berlin. The website is www. Institute-Microcirculation.com/en/basic-information. Here you will see a generalized discussion of our microcirculation.

At the bottom of that page is a video coming from his institute. He has one of the only facilities in the world with equipment capable of viewing live blood flow at the capillary level. You will see the video of someone with chronic stress. They looked at the blood flow in the colon of a twenty-seven-year-old athlete. Age was certainly not a factor, but chronic stress definitely takes its toll.

There is a therapy available that can influence the blood flow quite successfully. Because this device is presently going through Class II certification with the FDA, I cannot name the device in this book. However, in Europe it is registered as a Class II device, meaning recognized as effective for nine different circulation related conditions. If you would like further information about this, please email me at DTW@CET.com. I would be happy to provide additional information. It has been quite amazing to see changes take place in people's quality of life when they begin to experience the benefits of renewed increased microcirculation.

One area in which we have seen some significant synergistic response is when we have combined increased blood flow while doing syntonic light therapy (please see the syntonics chapter). To me, this makes a great deal of sense. If we can increase blood flow while doing the syntonic light therapy treatment, it should be quite helpful.

With the syntonics, one area we evaluate is a person's near-point functional visual field or their ability to detect awareness of a change in their peripheral vision with each eye when looking at a near-point distance.

We have had numerous patients where we measure their near-point functional visual field, and it will show significant constriction. We then do the syntonic light therapy while the patient is receiving the benefit of increased blood flow. Eight minutes later when we measure their near-point functional visual field, we will often see quite a noticeable increase in how soon they are able to detect the target coming into view from their peripheral vision. This has been particularly effective with a number of people with chronic stress who have seen significant changes within a matter of days. Before, it often could take several weeks before differences were observed.

I have noticed personally with this device that due to its ability to increase blood flow, it has been very helpful for both exercising and recovering from exercise. I really enjoy playing Ultimate Frisbee. The game involves quite a bit of running back and forth. Now at age sixty, I will take anything I can get to help me try to hang in there with the teenagers and young adult families we play with. After a couple of hours of Ultimate Frisbee, I feel it. From the use of this device, by increasing the blood flow, I have noticed a significant increase in my recovery time. I am not nearly as sore as I normally would be.

Additionally, jet lag has been pretty much eliminated when using the device while flying. Having the ability to improve blood flow while sitting for hours on a plane is so helpful. This last spring my wife and I were coming back from a tour in Israel and were up for about thirty-six hours, sleeping about five hours during that time. We arrived in Spokane, went to bed, and woke up at a normal time the next day and amazingly felt just fine. Another feature of the device is a patented sleep program which also is so helpful.

In addition to the sleep program, I will also use this device every morning. If it is going to be a morning of high-intensity interval training, I will use it for a few minutes right after I wake up and then do a ten- to fifteen-minute high-intensity interval training workout. I notice that it does allow me to increase the intensity of my workout during this time, no doubt due to the increased blood flow and oxygen-carrying capability that goes along with the increased blood flow.

Our whole extended family has found a number of benefits using this very simple yet profoundly effective device that is helping quality of life in so many ways. I look forward to my wife and I continuing to use it for the rest of our lives to help sustain blood flow the best we can. For more information, feel free to contact me.

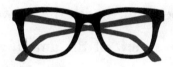

SURPRISING AND DISTURBING CAUSE OF RED, IRRITATED EYES

Occasionally, everyone will have red eyes or irritated, dry eyes. It is usually the result of spending too much time doing computer work, an environmental irritant, or not getting enough sleep. For those people who day after day have problems with irritated eyes, it can be extremely annoying.

There can be a multitude of factors. Nutrition and diet can be one. If a person has a particular sensitivity to foods or cosmetic products, that can be a source of irritation. In my practice, artificial sweetener consumption has been a notorious contributor for causing underlying eye irritation. It could be from the environment, like the humidity where you live. Do you live in the Sahara

Desert? Are you in a vehicle for many hours a day commuting with the heater or air conditioner on, which contributes to an extremely dry atmosphere? Is your workplace a source of very dry air?

Are your eyes red? Are they itchy? Do the eyelids themselves seem puffy, inflamed, or irritated? Do you have little flakes of dandruff-like tissue or collarets of mucous around the base of the eyelashes? If the environment is not the issue and if what you are taking into or putting onto your body is not an issue, what could be the cause of that irritation? Stay tuned, and let me tell you. I know you will not be thrilled with the answer.

First, let's do a brief overview of the amazing lacrimal, or tear, system, the eyelids, what all goes on, and a number of the structures involved with keeping the front part of our eye healthy.

The cornea, the clear window of the front part of our eye, has an absolutely amazing design. The cornea is made up of five layers of tissue. The individual cells are arranged and the layers spaced precisely the right distance apart to allow the visible light spectrum to pass through the cornea. The majority of bending of light to focus into the eye takes place at the corneal surface. Any disruption or inflammation to the cornea will cause swelling. This will decrease the clarity of vision as light begins to scatter.

Under an electron microscope, the top epithelial layer of the cornea looks like the surface of the moon. Many irregularities become visible under a high level of magnification. That is where the tear layer comes in because it is responsible for the crystal-clear focus of light that takes place at the corneal surface. The liquid layer fills in over the top of those microscopic irregularities to provide a clear bending of light.

Our tear film is composed of three main components. There is a mucin, or very thin, mucous component. It is closest to the top surface of the cornea. The epithelium has microvilli, or microscopic fingerlike projections that stick out and provide additional surface area for the mucin to be held against the epithelial cells. On top of that is a thin water layer. On top of that is a very thin oil film on the very top of the tear layer to decrease evaporation. If any of those main components are missing or in an improper ratio, problems can begin to arise.

From a dietary perspective, eating good fats (and being able to assimilate those fats) is an underlying foundational component to allow the body to have proper building blocks for a good-quality tear film base. Hydration would certainly be an additional factor. If the body is habitually dehydrated, it is going to be more difficult to have enough fluid for the tears to be in full production.

One not uncommon cause of repeated eye irritation can be due to what was just mentioned prior. At night, the major repair and regeneration of the corneal cells take place. The top layer of our cornea is replicated or replaced every seven to ten days.

At night, there is a lot of metabolic activity going on. If someone is chronically dehydrated, it is not uncommon to have part of the repair process end up sticking to the inside of the eyelid. When the person wakes in the morning and opens their eyes, some of the repair cells are pulled off similar to the way a Band-Aid would pull a scab off a wound on your knee. Microscopically, that opens up the corneal scratch or abrasion, so the next night it is trying to repair again. You can have that recurrent corneal abrasion happening night after night, leading to persistent eye irritation. Please keep in mind the natural ophthalmic gel drops which we have found have a high rate of success for helping that particular condition.

What if that is not the problem? What is another possibility I was alluding to in the first of this report? Jan Richard Bruenech, PhD, a professor of ocular anatomy and founding director of the biomedical research unit at the Buskerud and Vestfold University in Norway, presented some fascinating research of studies done looking at potential causes of red irritated eyes. He is a world-renowned anatomist, and he had some "eye-opening" microscope pictures of the different anatomical structures of the eyelid, the various glands in the eyelid that produce the fluids responsible for eye lubrication and tear preservation, and some up close and personal pictures of the most likely contributor to a significant number of red, itchy eyes.

At the Northwest Congress Optometric Extension meeting in Forest Grove, Oregon, at the end of February 2016, he was describing the incredible intricate design of the various structures in the eye among which are the mast cells, which are the cells that increase in quantity and size when there is an irritation contributing, which cause the body's inflammatory response to engage. They are responsible for the histamine production and release, which is part of the inflammatory response.

Further pictures were of the meibomian glands, which are the numerous glands in our eyelids that produce mucin for clinging onto those microvilli on the cornea. There was a very thin epithelial layer of tissue that lines these meibomian glands. Right next door are the sebaceous glands which produce the oil, the top layer that decreases the evaporation of the tears. Those are produced at the base of the eyelashes, or the follicles of the eyelashes.

Studies in Norway looking at over one-hundred fifty people in various age groups found that starting around age thirty, approximately 50 percent of people had in their eyelash follicles this irritant contributor to inflammation. By age fifty, it was approximately 75 percent. Above age sixty-five, it was more than 90 percent of people who had Demodex. Those are lovely little parasitic mites that live in or near hair follicles of most mammals. That includes us. Creepy, isn't it?

He went on to describe the life cycle of the Demodex. There is no need to go into details. Just know it is disgusting. He mentioned that these little parasites are quite tough. They can live for many hours, almost up to a day, under a microscope light before expiring. They are not light-lovers, so they try to get away from light.

One of the most common treatments for blepharitis or eyelid irritation is antibiotics. Unfortunately, antibiotics do not bother the Demodex very much. Also, since they are hiding down in the eyelash follicles, it is more difficult for any topical medication to get to the site of where they are hiding.

To further add to the word picture, a person could have up to fifteen Demodex per eyelash. The diameter of the Demodex is almost exactly the same size as the little pockets in the hair follicle where they fit, as Dr. Bruenech says, "nicely like a cork". (This is not getting any better, is it?)

Tea tree oil is one product that has been found to be effective against the Demodex.

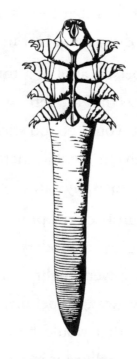

Demodex

However, it is quite irritating to the eye, and it is quite painful to apply. There are commercial available products which have that as part of the ingredients and have been shown effective for treatment.

There is one other option which is very nontoxic and does not sting, though it may be slightly sticky. That is the Manuka honey from New Zealand. Manuka honey has several health benefits. It is recommended that one use Manuka honey that has an MGO, which is the amount of methylglyoxal content, of four hundred or more. Honey has a number of medicinal benefits and certainly is worth consideration.

When we think of a romantic evening, we think of candlelight, low lights, and soft music. The Demodex are not that much different from us (although I do not know about the music part). In the evening when we go to sleep, the Demodex find that love is in the air. That is when they become most active. (It is still disgusting, isn't it?)

If a person applies a thin film of Manuka honey along the base of their eyelashes as they are getting ready to go to bed, and they could use a tiny bit of water if it would be too sticky to get on, this can be very helpful. The honey, to some extent, would increase the odds of potentially allowing some of the Demodex to asphyxiate.

The antibacterial properties of the Manuka honey can be very helpful for decreasing any secondary bacterial infections. Certainly your eyelids will be a little sticky every night, but in the morning you just use warm water to rinse the honey away. Hopefully, you will wash away the honey as well as the lovely Demodex that would be within the honey. As their lifespan is two to three weeks, you will want to continue nightly application for one month.

There are a number of advantages of this method. First is cutting down the unnecessary use of antibiotics, which contributes to antibiotic-resistant bacteria formation. It is much more likely to get to the underlying cause of the itching and inflammation. It is doing that without any irritants to the sensitive eye tissue. For those of you who have chronic red, irritated eyes, I recommend you give this a try. It definitely puts a new meaning to the phrase, "Goodnight and sweet dreams."

CONCLUSION

"Breathtaking!" is still a word that comes to mind when I think about the incredible attributes of the amazingly designed visual system. So powerful a sense it is, having five times the input to the brain of any other of our senses. Yet also how subtle but profound can be its influence on our daily lives.

My wish is that this book has given you some additional information that you can use to look into helping you or a loved one with visual difficulties.

I think you will agree, "There certainly is more than meets the eye!" and if your eyes could talk, they certainly would have a lot to say!

D. Todd Wylie, OD, FCOVD